Happy
Sleeping
Baby

Your Guide for Sleep Success

Courtney Landin

Printed in the United States of America
Publisher's Cataloging-in-Publication data
Landin, Courtney.
Cover photo: Shutterstock images
Graphic Design: Katarina Lapidoth/Lapidoth Design
Images in content: p. 9 Karin Boo, p. 13 Getty Images, p. 90 Jessica Hanlon
unsplash.com – p. 37 David Mao, p. 50 Jason Sung, p. 54 Minnie Zhou,
p. 70 Picsea, p. 72 Kevin Liang, p. 79 Noah Silliman, p. 94 Yeimy Oliver,
p. 105 Picsea, p. 135 Jonathan Borba, p. 142 Mahmud Ahsan, p. 155 Janko Ferlic,
p. 175 Thiago Cerqueira, p. 186 S L, p. 193 Charles Deluvio, p. 202 Minnie Zhou,
p. 204 Callim Hill
Shutterstock images – p. 21, 66, 93, 99, 120, 164
Illustrator Bedtime routine chart: Yandeh Sallah

Happy Sleeping Baby: Your Guide for Sleep Success/Courtney Landin
ISBN 978-91-519-8212-0
First Edition

Content

Forward   7
About the author   9
What to expect from this book   14
How to use this book   18
Safety checklist   22
Safe sleeping conditions   23
Postpartum depression/anxiety   25

Chapter 1 – Understanding sleep   27
    What is sleep?   27
    Sleep stages   28
    Sleeping through the night   29
    Sleep stages at night   30
    Why does light or dark matter for sleep?   33
    Why is sleep important?   35

Chapter 2 – Happy sleep basics   39
    Week 1   39
    Before you begin   40
    Sleepy cues   41
    Awake windows   42
    Avoid over-tiredness   44
    Room environment   45
    What's all the hype about white noise?   46
    Sleep props   46
    Your sleeping phrases   50
    Routines   52
    Naps   58
    How to wake your baby from a nap   60
    Napping-on-the-go   60
    Reducing nap (and eliminating naps)   61

Is your baby ready to drop a nap?   62
Three options to drop a nap   63
Setting up bedtime   64
Eliminate screen time   64
The last step ... falling asleep   70
What about co-sleeping?   72
Setting up for sleep check-list   73

Chapter 3 – Factors that affect sleep   75
What are regressions and milestones?   75
Nightmare or night terror?   78
Stress levels   81
Emotional regulation (handling emotions)   85
Learning to self-soothe   87
Consistency   92
Sensitivity and temperament   92
Talk, talk, talk!!   98
Using sign language   100
Pacifiers   101
Developmental tips to help sleep   104
Teething   106
Your relationship after baby   108
Sometimes it's difficult to fall back to sleep   115

Chapter 4 – Schedules and development by age   117
The first 8 weeks   118
What does the fourth trimester mean for you?   123
Crying – is it colic?   125
Baby sounds   130
2 to 3 months (8 – 12 weeks)   132
Does an early bedtime matter?   133
3 – 6 months (12 – 24 weeks)   137
6 – 8 months (24 – 32 weeks)   144
8 – 12 months (32 – 48 weeks)   149
13 – 18 months   156
2 – 5 years   161

Chapter 5 – Steps towards more sleep   167
    What is sleep training?   167
    The three main baby sleep training methods 168
    Weeks 2 and 3   170
    Your sleep goals   174
    Happy sleep methods   176
    Day 1 and nights 1 through 4   177
    Crying   179
    Night waking   179
    What you might see   181
    Naptime – beginning on day 2   182
    Night 5 through 8   184
    Night 9 through 12   187
    Night 13 and 14   189
    Happy sleep and beyond   190
    Sleep trouble checklist   192

Appendix   195
    Setting up for sleep checklist   195
    Sleep and nap chart   195
    Sleep logs   196
    Bedtime routine   197
    Hold & help sleep plan cheat sheet   199
    Fading sleep plan cheat sheet   201
    Leave & check sleep plan cheat sheet   203

References   208
Thank you   216

People who say they've slept like a baby, have never had one.

#mumlife

Forward

Congratulations on making a big step towards figuring out your baby's sleep and also getting closer to sleeping through the night again. Parenting is the hardest, yet most rewarding job there is! A baby brings such joy to a family, but can also bring a lot of sleepless nights. The newborn and toddler years can be difficult stages that can affect you and your family's life due to lack of sleep. Luckily, you've found *Happy Sleeping Baby – Your Guide for Sleep Success* and by reading it, you will gain valuable knowledge about helping your baby (and you!) sleep better.

The concept of teaching a baby to sleep may sound a little strange to you as a parent. Surely, a child should enjoy and benefit from natural sleep rather than be trained or taught. That's what I thought in the beginning too! Then I had a baby who needed help understanding when it was time to sleep and what that feeling meant in her body. The thing about "training" your child is that it can actually help them, and you, to get the right amount of restful sleep. It's a way of protecting your baby and keeping them healthy and happy. *Training or practicing healthy sleep habits is no different than your baby learning how to eat or crawl on their own. Both take time, practice, and patience.*

While you go through this book, one of the most important things to remember is that every child will go through the same developmental stages, but every stage can and will look different from child to child. There are personality and temperament factors to take into account, as well. What works in one home may not work in another and making some adjustments to the recommendations will be fine!

Sleep training doesn't always have the best reputation, but it is simply a way for you to help your child understand how to sleep so he or she can get the rest they need. If your child still seems reluctant to sleep for longer periods, do not worry. As I mentioned earlier, every child is different. Your baby may simply need to be a little older before he or she can begin to understand how to sleep for longer stretches. It's normal for babies to wake up during the night and you'll understand why in Chapter 1.

The purpose of writing this book is to save you the time of trying to find the right method, schedule, and routines; not to mention save you countless hours of reading and questioning what you need to achieve what you are trying to do. Through personal experience, education, and numerous hours of working with parents and their babies, I have put together information and guidance that works wonders in helping babies and young children to achieve happy sleep! This book is focused on educating you about sleep for your child's whole life and finding a solution for different stages of his or her life. I get so frustrated when books are only filled with testimonials of how well a method worked for other parents and all you want is to figure out how to help *your* child sleep, not get a vague explanation of what to do on page 303 that leaves you wondering about what's next or if you're doing it correctly.

Sleep is a process and this book will empower you as a parent to understand the basics of sleep and help your child develop healthy sleep habits and skills for life. Remember, training, learning, or practicing healthy sleep habits is no different than your baby learning how to eat or crawl on her own. Both take time, practice, and patience! Another important point I want to emphasize is that there isn't just one way for all children. I offer many different options if you find that one isn't working for you. Most importantly is that consistency creates security and success for your children, so give them those to have sleep success!

Throughout the book I'll use either he or she to ease reading.

About the author and her sleep struggle

I'm Courtney, a Family Health Coach focusing on exercise, nutrition and sleep to help your family thrive. One of my main focus areas is infant and child sleep because it is an important aspect for the whole family to feel amazing. I know because we suffered through months of sleepless nights.

My search for sleep guidance began a few months after my daughter was born. I honestly thought I had experienced enough sleep deprivation after being in the military and also traveling through numerous time zones as an athlete that I thought I was ready for what was to come.

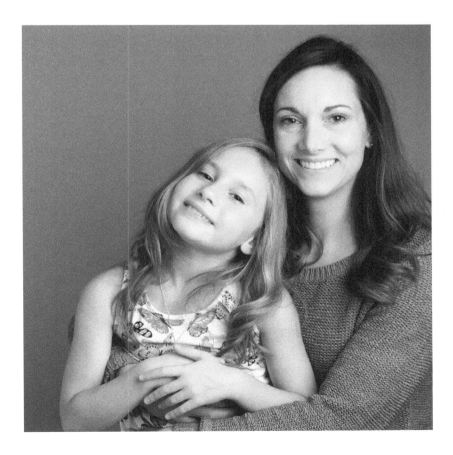

I was prepared for sleepless nights and also thought I had read quite a lot before she was born, so I knew what to do – but I had no idea what was ahead of me. Everyone I talked to with babies said they slept and that it's boring to have a newborn! So, silly me, I decided to continue studying for my MBA assuming I'd have so much time to study. Well, after eight months, I was still waking up every two hours or less at night and truly struggling during the days. My husband and I started to understand why sleep deprivation is a form of torture. It sounds funny, I know, but it definitely did not seem funny at the time, as I'm sure you understand! Our little girl screamed when she was put down and therefore, she lived on me day and night. I didn't understand why she wasn't sleeping like a baby should.

Whenever I stopped moving, sat down, or finally fell asleep myself, she immediately woke up and started screaming again. It was a nightmare that was totally overwhelming, not to mention physically and mentally exhausting. The other mamas I knew were not having these issues and I also felt like I was failing as a parent. I was so sleep deprived that I was seeing black spots, I thought I was seeing a cat in our apartment (we don't have a cat), my anxiety was through the roof, and I was not enjoying being a mama, which made me even sadder. Both my husband and I were at our wits end and in need of sleep.

We had some relief around six months old when, after many trips to the doctor where I was looked at like I was crazy, I was told that "babies cry and it's just a phase." We found out that she had a dairy and peanut allergy, which contributed to her discomfort and general fussiness. She wasn't allergic to sleep; she was allergic to dairy and peanuts! Never doubt your parental instinct if something "doesn't feel right!" After this discovery and after eliminating dairy and peanuts (which I had been eating a lot of, goodbye Reese peanut butter cups!), she was much happier, but we soon realized that we had a sleeping issue due to us constantly trying to provide her comfort for many months. My daughter had developed a dependency on being held and rocked to sleep, only for her to wake when put down. *These methods are not wrong and I encourage you to do this in the beginning,* but it becomes extremely tiring when a child becomes dependent on these in order to be put to sleep and stay asleep after many months. At six months old, she didn't know what a bed was or what it was like to lay down in one! It was time for a change because my back was killing me and I was exhausted!

In hopes of change, I scoured the Internet for information and ultimately found sleep methods that worked! After a few months of perseverance and making some changes to the sleep advice I was using, we found our rhythm. Of course, we still had our 'off' days and that's only human, but on the whole we all enjoy peaceful and restful sleep 99% of the time. Not only that, but if you had told me back at the start of our sleep journey that our daughter would lean towards her crib when she wanted to go to sleep, I would never have believed you. But that is what she did!

What I learned helped my family to regain proper sleep and I became passionate about learning how I could help other struggling families. Sleep is important for our children, but sleep deprivation is also a serious matter for us as parents. My goal of writing this book is to help other parents understand that there are things you can do to help your child sleep, but also to understand the many different aspects involved. You are not failing as a parent if your baby isn't sleeping through the night at six weeks old or even at one year! There are factors that can help your baby, and you, sleep better!

My sleep education

My interest in sleep began before I had my daughter. I was an Olympic athlete competing for the United States (under my maiden name of Courtney Zablocki) and for 16 years, I raced down an icy track competing in the sport of Luge. I traveled the world competing in World Cups, multiple World Championship races, and then in the 2002 and 2006 Olympic Games. During this time, I started learning how important sleep is to rejuvenate the mind and body. While I was an athlete, I also joined the Colorado National Guard and went through 18 weeks of military basic training. This was a tough test of physical and mental ability while sleep deprived. But it wasn't until I had little Taylor that I fully understood the meaning of sleep deprivation and the importance of sleep. I would have gladly gone back to basic training when she was a newborn! Man, do I wish I had slept more when I was younger!

After retiring from my sport in 2010, I joined the business world but quickly realized I missed the athletic life because sitting at a desk was not for me. I then became a personal trainer and a Pre- and Postnatal Corrective Exercise Specialist because I was fascinated by the body during pregnancy, and also saw that women need more guidance on how to take care of their bodies during this stage of life.

After suffering from countless sleepless nights and finally figuring out my daughter's sleep struggle, I decided to train as a sleep consultant and thereafter completed a certification program to understand how to help parents with their child's sleep (as you probably are figuring out, sleep is a hot topic among parents). From there, I continued to take courses on Infant Mental Health through the Infant Mental Health Promotion program based in Toronto, Canada, and later completed a Certified Sleep Science Coach program. I also continue to educate myself on current research around sleep issues both for adults and babies, as well as child development. With all of this information, I created my Happy Sleep program, which I believe is the most comprehensive sleep program that combines sleep education, mental health and developmental health information, along with sleep techniques that actually work. Helping infants and children sleep better is my passion and I

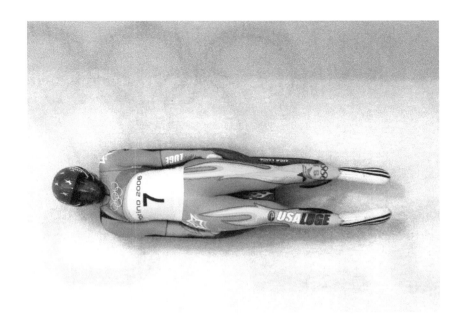

continue to keep up to date with current studies on sleep and development because sleep is such a critical part of our health, no matter what age.

I want to share this knowledge with you and help you through the hard, sleepless nights that come with being a parent. Yes, some parts are difficult phases to get through and there isn't a solution for everything, but the majority of the time it doesn't have to be a struggle. There are aspects you can change to help you and your child get the sleep you both need! Enjoy the sleep journey and I'm so happy that you are reading this book!

Here's to healthy and happy families!
~*Courtney*

Join me on Instagram and Facebook at
@HappySleepingBaby
or find more information at
HappySleepingBaby.com

What to expect from this book

First of all, I have some news that I'm going to break to you. Here it is: your sleep will not be the same as a parent. Don't expect to sleep the same as when you did before kids. At least not for the first several years because kids will wake up occasionally! There, I said it.

I'm not saying this to make you throw your hands in the air and think there's nothing you can do, but it's important to understand that sleep just won't be the same for a while. You'll be woken up more, woken up at different times than you'd like, and there's more mental and physical energy being used as a parent, so you're constantly tired. But the good news is that you can start implementing healthier habits and reduce the amount of sleep challenges you confront as much as possible and that's what we'll be doing in this book.

I know that you are tired and want your child to sleep better *right now*, but please understand that sleep is a process and also a puzzle. All of the puzzle pieces need to be in place to help your child sleep better.

Keep in mind that making changes can take anywhere from three weeks to three months depending on how quickly you make changes or would like to make changes, along with other factors that may come into play, such as illness or traveling.

This book is different in that it helps you understand sleep and how it works in our bodies. It also allows you to be your child's guide through the process. Change can be hard, especially when your child may not understand why something they are used to doing is changing, even if it is for healthier ways! Yet, by guiding your child through the changes, they are able to learn and know you are there for them. During this process, you will ultimately be able to help your child, and yourself, get better sleep.

Let's also talk about what sleep training really means since the term doesn't have the best reputation. Basically, sleep training can mean whatever you want it to mean. Are you okay with your child crying or would you prefer to assist your child as much as possible? Both are "sleep training" because it's helping your child learn a skill and that takes time. Don't think that sleep training is bad! In fact, you are being an *amazing* parent because you are helping your child learn a healthy and important skill for life, while also giving yourself a very important aspect that you need as well. *Do not* have sleep training guilt about teaching your child an important skill either! This will be a skill they retain for the rest of their life.

This book is based on principles that focus on:
- developing an emotionally healthy child
- nurturing connections
- providing a secure attachment
- responding with sensitivity
- practicing positive discipline while providing healthy boundaries for children
- providing balance in personal and family life

This gives your child guidance, but also skills on how to help handle their emotions around sleep and daily life. This book will provide you with knowledge for your child's development and help them navigate learning their new skill of sleeping.

During the next several weeks, we'll be working on improving your child's sleep and although many of you may see improvements in just a week, many of you may not. The reason that there isn't a one-size-fits-all type of book or advice is because sleep takes work and your child is a human with his own feelings, wants, and needs, but children also have developmental stages that affect sleep. You can expect that this book will give you a better understanding of how to help your child establish healthy sleep habits for their whole life, to see improvements in their sleep, and know how to help your child sleep much better.

Watch out for sleep advice that claims there will be no crying or that your child will sleep through the night within three nights or that you won't ever have another sleep struggle. It's a marketing scam and not realistic. This is what gives us parents guilt, shame, and anxiety that our child isn't able to make changes that quickly.

I also want you to understand that there isn't one way that works for everyone and it's the reason there is so much contradictory information on what to do about sleep! There is no perfect approach that is for all families and this book offers parent-assisted approaches to offer you solutions for your child during their ups and downs.

There are other factors that affect sleep and will determine the amount of time and affect this will take such as, personalities and temperaments of both you and your child. Also know that this process can take a little time. There's no simple magic trick or cure to get you there, but what you will learn are tools to understand your child better and also make you a better parent because of that. Parenting is a roller-coaster that will always have ups and downs, even with sleep. You will learn a lot in the following weeks and the best thing that you will learn is that this isn't just a one-time use kind of program. You will be able to apply these tools throughout your child's life and you are giving them a gift of healthy sleep habits along the way.

I'm also not going to sugar coat this process. It will take work and it will seem like it gets worse before it gets better, but if you are consistent then you will see changes! If other books or advice offer you a solution that will begin working that night, then be hesitant about it and, I'll say it again, know it's a marketing scam! There is no overnight cure that takes minimal work. But I'll guide you through the changes you need to make to see lasting improvements. The important part of this journey is to start with the end goal in mind and be consistent!

Sleep success may look different for your family than others, so remember that there is no comparison or right way for your family to go about it. Some parents want to work towards zero wake-ups as soon as possible, while others are fine with a wake up until their child is two years old. Remember, what you decide is right for your family is what's successful.

How to use this book

Keep in mind that changes may take between three weeks to three months depending on the rate at which you make changes, would like to make changes, or other factors that may come into play, such as illness, development leaps, moving, or traveling.

Making changes will also depend on your child's personality, temperament, age, developmental stage, and your parenting style. Also keep in mind that what you had planned to do or how to be as a parent may change depending on your child's personality. Here's a quick overview of what to expect in each chapter.

Chapter 1

What is sleep

Chapter 1 helps you understand how sleep works and is an important aspect to understanding that sleep is a puzzle that must be figured out. It's a short read that offers you great insight on why we are making some of these changes. If you'd rather skip the background information and get started right away, begin with Chapter 2 and come back to Chapter 1 after you've started.

Chapter 2

Week 1

Within chapter 2, you'll be putting many pieces of the sleep puzzle together to set the groundwork for sleep success. This will include Week 1; beginning to make sleep changes for your child. These steps are great to begin at any age but you must begin with these steps, otherwise you will struggle more than necessary when continuing on to make changes for sleep. There is a lot covered in this chapter and it may take longer than a week to complete, so don't be afraid to take your time. Often,

I've had parent's work on these tasks and see small improvements in just a few days.

You'll continue onto Weeks 2 and 3 in Chapter 5, but in the meantime as you work on Chapter 2, you can read Chapters 3 and 4 to learn more about your child.

Within different sections of Chapter 2, you'll find *Sleep Tasks* for you to complete that help you put together what works for your family and helps you understand your child's sleep. This is helping to build your sleep puzzle for your family!

Chapter 2 is the meat of this book. The hard work goes on in this chapter to help you avoid moving on to Chapter 5. Yes, you read that correctly. I don't want you to read part of this book if you don't have to! Now, in some cases (depending on your child's age, temperament, and sleep prop) you will have to move onto Chapter 5, but do your best to use Chapter 2 to set up for sleep success first and work on as much as possible here.

Chapter 3

Development and more

This chapter will cover sleep regressions, milestones, temperaments, stress, development leaps, and educational tips to help your baby communicate with you. It will help you understand many of the road bumps you may experience and also help you and your child develop ways to understand each other better.

Chapter 4

Information by age ranges

Within this chapter, you will read about what to expect for your child's age and general nap schedules according to their age. You'll also notice that developmental aspects by age are covered here so you can understand your child better and the changes they are going through on a regular basis. You'll use Chapter 4 a lot and it will be useful as your child grows and changes.

Chapter 5

Weeks 3 & 4

This chapter will guide you through three weeks of different types of sleep training approaches. You'll start with the one that suits your family best. I've worked with many families where these outlines work great and have made many adjustments over the years to make sure these can be adapted for your needs.

I want to emphasise that no matter which option you choose, all of the puzzle pieces need to be in place for sleep to work and know that you aren't failing if it doesn't always work right away! Some changes may take time to see results.

Appendix

In this section you'll find sleep log templates, a cheat sheet for your sleep plan, a bedtime routine chart, space to write your own plan, and any other notes you find helpful along the way. This section is your tool to make your sleep plan work for your family.

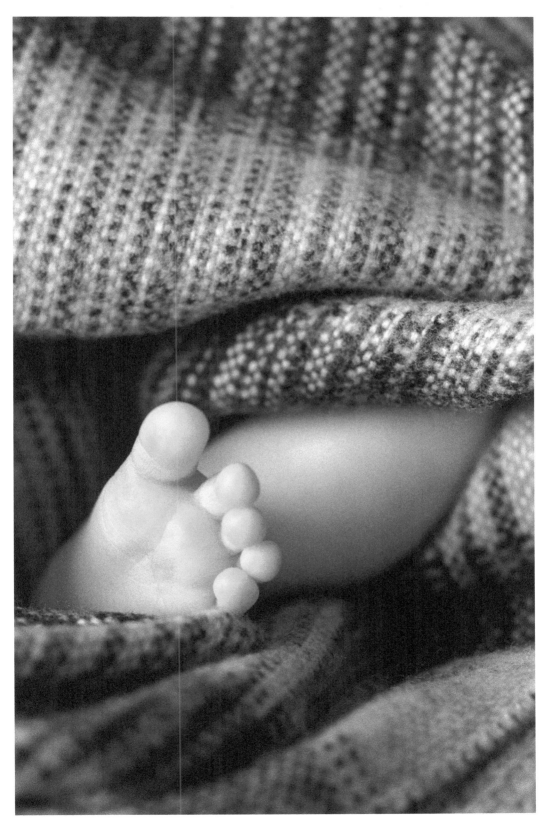

Safety checklist

Before you begin making sleep changes, please complete this checklist and contact your doctor if you have any concerns.

Does your baby snore or breathe heavily through his mouth?

While it is common to breathe heavier when sick, heavy breathing, mouth breathing, or snoring should not happen on a regular basis. This could be a sign your child has difficulties breathing and it is affecting the ability to fall asleep or to stay asleep. If you answer yes, please check with your doctor before moving on to Chapter 5.

Does your baby arch his or her back, seem uncomfortable in a car seat or seated position, or throw up often?

If your baby regularly arches his back, throws up often, or is uncomfortable in a seated position, it could indicate GI or reflux issues. It is common for babies to have some form of reflux as their food pipe (esophagus) connects the mouth to the stomach and is not fully developed until about a year old, but some babies have issues with this even though it's normal. This could interfere with your child's ability to calm down or feel comfortable. If you answer yes, speak with your doctor if you think this is an issue and avoid the positions your child is uncomfortable in; such as car seats or positions that put pressure on the stomach.

Does your child have constipation, loose stool, or mucus in her diaper?

While it is common for babies to have different types of stool as their food changes, it can indicate intestinal irritation, food sensitivity, or an allergy. Notice if some foods cause your child to feel uncomfortable or become cranky after eating and speak with your doctor if you think this is a problem. This can cause difficulties in feeling comfortable or settling for sleep if your child has tummy issues.

Does your baby have skin rashes or eczema?

Skin rashes can indicate a food allergy or sensitivity or too dry climate. Babies often have sensitivities or allergies to foods such as milk protein, nuts, eggs, or other food items. This can cause difficulties in feeling comfortable or settling for sleep if your child is uncomfortable or itchy. Check with your doctor for more advice if you think this is an issue for your child.

I've included these questions to help you understand any underlying issues for your child. *If your child has one of the above, it can affect his ability to self-soothe or feel calm. Trying to make sleep changes while your child is uncomfortable or unable to calm himself will only result in a struggle.* Contact your doctor if you have any concerns about any of the above issues.

Safe sleeping conditions

According to the American Academy of Pediatrics, experts agree that putting a baby to sleep or down for a nap on his or her back is the safest position, as side-sleeping has a higher risk for SIDS than back sleeping.

Other reports have found the following factors also increase the risk for SIDS:

- soft surfaces
- loose bedding
- overheating with too many blankets
- stomach sleeping on soft bedding
- smoking by the mother
- poor prenatal care and prematurity

Since the American Academy of Pediatrics (AAP) made the "back-to-sleep" recommendation in 1992, the SIDS rate has dropped more than 50%. Back sleeping also appears to be safer for other reasons as well. Despite common conceptions, there is no evidence that babies are more likely to vomit or spit up while sleeping on their back. In fact, choking may be more likely in the prone position.

A task force of The U.S. Consumer Product Safety Commission, the AAP, and the National Institute of Child Health and Human Development offer the following recommendations for infant bedding:

- Place your baby on his or her back on a firm, tight-fitting mattress in a crib that meets current safety standards.
- Remove pillows, quilts, comforters, sheepskins, stuffed toys, and other soft products from the crib. Also remove any soft, pillow-like crib bumpers.
- Consider using a sleep sack as an alternative to blankets with no other covering.
- If using a blanket, put your baby with his or her feet at the foot of the crib. Tuck a thin blanket around the crib mattress, only as far as the baby's chest.
- Make sure your baby's head remains uncovered during sleep.
- Do not place your baby on a waterbed, sofa, soft mattress, pillow, or other soft surface to sleep.
- Offer your newborn a pacifier at sleep times, but don't force the baby to take it. Some studies have shown a lower rate of SIDS among newborn babies who use pacifiers.

The AAP and the US Department of Health and Human Services recommends that parents room share, but not bed share. The report advises the following:

- Parents should consider placing the infant's crib near their bed for more convenient breastfeeding and parent contact for the first six months to one year.
- Infants can be brought into the parents' bed for feedings and comforting, but should be returned to their own crib for sleep.
- Infants should not bed share with others, including adults and siblings or other children. Twins and other multiples should sleep separately.
- Smoking and the use of substances, such as drugs or alcohol, that may impair parents' ability to awaken greatly increase the risk of SIDS and suffocation with bed sharing.

While the true cause of SIDS is unknown, these recommendations can help reduce your baby's risk and give him a safe sleeping environment.

Postpartum depression/anxiety

Having a baby is a life changing experience and it's normal for you and/ or your partner to have symptoms of depression or anxiety. It's common to feel tired, have trouble sleeping, have a change in appetite, feel more worried or a little low, or have mood changes after having a baby.

Postpartum depression or anxiety are more intense and last longer than generalized anxiety or depression. Symptoms include a depressed mood, loss of pleasure, feelings of worthlessness, hopelessness, helplessness, thoughts of death or suicide, thoughts of hurting someone else, or feeling overly worried about your baby.

If you have had high levels of stress either during pregnancy or after bringing your baby home, keep in mind you are at a higher risk of symptoms. Plus, not sleeping enough increases your chance of depression and anxiety. You are not alone if you feel this way. If you are concerned or experience any of the symptoms above, contact your healthcare provider for help during this time. Talk with your partner or reach out to friends or family for extra help at home. Having a baby is a huge life change and you don't have to do it alone!

If you are struggling with postpartum depression, begin with Chapter 2 to start developing healthy sleep habits for your baby to increase the chances of getting better sleep for yourself, as well. More sleep can reduce feelings of depression and anxiety. Remember, your life is changing and it's okay to have different emotions during this time. Parenting isn't full of rainbows and unicorns all the time. It's perfectly normal to feel low, question your ability to be a parent, or not enjoy every second. Reach out for others to help you! *It's okay to ask for help.*

Understanding sleep

What is sleep?

Our first step to helping your child sleep is to put into place some simple items that work with their bodies so that sleep can happen more naturally. One important part of this is to first understand how our bodies sleep and what exactly sleep is.

Sleep is a 24-hour cyclical process that is affected by what we do during the day. We have two systems within our bodies that regulate sleep, which are great to know because it will help you to understand why it's important to set your child up for sleep.

CIRCADIAN BIOLOGICAL CLOCK (RHYTHM) – This is a 24-hour rhythm in your body that dips and rises at different times of the day to regulate the timing of sleepiness and wakefulness. Your brain communicates this rhythm to every part of your brain and every organ in your body. The sleepiness we experience during these circadian dips will be less intense if we have had sufficient sleep, and more intense when we are sleep deprived. The circadian rhythm also causes us to feel more alert at certain points of the day, even if we have been awake for hours. For adults, we generally experience a dip around 1 pm – 3 pm. Contrary to what you may think, it's not lunch that makes you feel sleepy, it's your circadian rhythm and a bit of sleep pressure, which you'll learn about below!

This rhythm is so important in our bodies that it doesn't just time when we feel sleepy, it also sets our preferences for eating, drinking, moods, emotions, body temperature, and release of hormones.

SLEEP PRESSURE – Our need for sleep accumulates in the body throughout the day and signals that it is time to sleep. This is called "sleep pressure" and this feeling accumulates in the body due to a hormone that builds up in the brain called adenosine. If this hormone isn't flushed out of the brain, it accumulates to induce sleepiness the next time your circadian rhythm dips, just like that midday dip, for example. This increases tiredness and causes the body to fall asleep, if there's the opportunity.

These two systems work together during the day and night to regulate when we should sleep and when we should be awake. While there's a lot more that goes into how our bodies sleep, now you understand the basic principles of what sleep is in the body and the terms you'll read within the book.

Sleep stages

We all know we need sleep, but what exactly is sleep? Do we fall off into a different world and always wake up rested? Why are you more tired when you wake up one morning but feel ready to go the next morning, even if you've had the same number of hours? Research shows that sleep is an active part of our life and important for growth, learning, memory, and proper functioning, not only for babies but for adults too. Sleep restores our brains and bodies from the day's events and learning. To understand sleep better, let's break down how our bodies go through this process.

AS ADULTS, our bodies go through sleep cycles of around 90 – 120 minutes. Newborn babies have a cycle of around 30 – 60 minutes until about 4 months of age when their cycles transition closer to an adult's sleep cycle. We have different stages of sleep too, which I'm sure you are aware of if you've watched your baby sleep, but let's go over them in more detail.

FOR NEWBORN babies until around four months of age, the sleep cycle is more evenly divided between REM and NREM sleep. A newborn's sleep cycle looks like this:

- When a baby first falls asleep, they go into active sleep, which is very similar to REM (rapid eye movement) sleep for adults (see description on the following page). During this stage, babies are also more likely to wake up. A newborn will spend about 50% of his or her sleeping cycles in this stage, as opposed to an adult, with only 20%.

- About halfway through a sleep cycle, the baby falls into quiet sleep, which is characterized by slower, rhythmic breathing, less movement, and no eyelid fluttering. Quiet sleep is the end of the sleep cycle, which means that the baby will either wake up or return to active sleep.

Newborns will cycle through these two stages of sleep until about four months of age when their body will transition to sleep cycles similar to that of an adult. This is typically the four month sleep regression stage!

Sleeping through the night

Let's squash one myth and one I wish I had known when I was a new parent. In the medical world, "sleeping through the night" means *five* hours of uninterrupted sleep. Not a blissful 12 where you all wake up refreshed and ready for the day. Sleeping through the night is defined from 12:00 am – 5:00 am during the first 8 weeks of life; *five* hours where your baby sleeps without waking you. Now, this doesn't mean that your baby doesn't wake up, it just means that he slept without waking you. This is also true as your baby gets older. They may wake up, but you aren't aware of it.

Sleep stages at night

Sleep seems like quite a simple concept, but it's more than just being awake and being asleep. There are two stages of sleep, NREM (non-rapid eye movement) and REM (rapid eye movement), that we go through during the course of a night. Completing each of these sleep stages is important for the body and brain to recover, develop, and grow.

Generally, it takes most adults around 10 to 20 minutes to fall asleep. Of course, there are certain nights this time may be more or less. It's also important to note that if you fall asleep too quickly or if it takes beyond a half hour most nights to drift into dreamland, there may be an underlying issue to consider. If you tend to fall asleep quickly, you may be sleep deprived. If you have trouble falling asleep you may want to look at what you are doing before bedtime, such as looking at t.v. or your phone or how much caffeine you drink during the day.

When we sleep, we typically pass through each of the following stages for about 5 – 15 minutes each before moving on to the next. The sleep stages look like this:

THE FIRST STAGE (LIGHT SLEEP, NREM) is the lightest stage of NREM (non-rapid eye movement) sleep and is characterized by little eye movement. It's generally a stage of drowsiness where you are still slightly aware that you are awake and can be easily woken. Muscle tone relaxes and brain wave activity starts to decrease.

THE SECOND STAGE (DEEPER LIGHT SLEEP, NREM) of sleep is actually the first stage of NREM, whereby it is a little harder to be woken or aroused during stage 2. Brain waves continue to slow, body temperature decreases, and heart rate slows. You start to feel heavy in your body and if woken at this stage, you will know that you were drifting off to sleep.

THE THIRD SLEEP STAGE (DEEP SLEEP, NREM) is known as deep NREM sleep and is the most restorative of all of the stages, consisting mostly delta (slow) waves. Awakenings in this stage are rare. It is also the stage where sleepwalking, sleep talking, and night terrors occur. Breathing slows, heart rate and blood pressure decrease, and the body is very still during this stage. If you are woken, it would take some shaking and very loud talking to get you out of your slumber. You would feel very groggy and it would take a while to actually feel awake when woken during deep sleep. Deep sleep is the stage that growth hormone is released into the body for repair and recovery. This stage also helps boost immunity, regulates blood pressure, and repairs muscles and tissues. Deep sleep tends to happen more towards the first half of the night but if your body is trying to make up for sleep, then there will be some deep sleep later in the night, as well.

THE RAPID EYE MOVEMENT (REM) STAGE is most common for dreams. We actually dream in other stages, but these are the dreams we remember and are in color. Eyes move rapidly from side to side and brain waves are much more active than in stage two or three. Unlike stage three, awakening can occur more easily in REM and often leaves one feeling groggy and overly tired. Your body will make small movements, noises, or twitch during this stage. If you wake up during REM, you will be aware of your dream. This stage is when our brains move information from short to long term memory, and tends to happen during the second half of the night.

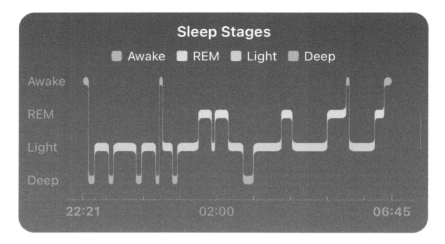

Generally, this is what it looks like when our bodies cycle through the sleep stages at night.

Notice that deep sleep is more towards the first part of the night and REM sleep is more towards the second part of the night. This is because our bodies reduce the production of melatonin partway through the night. This is also the reason you may notice your baby wakes more the second half of the night and that you have a harder time falling asleep again.

Although sleep loss is kind of inevitable when you have a newborn, it's still important to prioritize getting as much extra sleep as possible because your body needs it to function, have a healthy immune system, and for your brain to work! Sadly, we can't make up for lost sleep, but our bodies are smart and will go into longer stages of deep and NREM sleep for the first couple of nights, if you are able to sleep longer, and then a few days later your brain will have more REM sleep to even things out.

LET'S RECAP SLEEP STAGES

Four sleep stages = one sleep cycle
Adults and older children = 90 to 120-minute cycles
Babies under four months = 30 to 60-minute cycles

Adults can cycle from REM sleep to stage one and then stage two again without much of a problem. We are used to these wake ups and they don't tend to bother us much during the night. We tend to have five to six sleep cycles each night, while children will have six or more. Babies, who wake up after one cycle or throughout the night, generally have something that wakes them up or they are accustomed to having some sort of help to fall asleep. They don't know how to transition from stage one to stage two and beyond again and this is very normal for babies!

Why do you wake up rested one morning and groggy the next?

There are many factors to this answer but one of the main factors depends on when you woke up and during which sleep stage you were in. If you wake up naturally or right after a dream, you'll feel rested and ready for the day. If you wake up during deep sleep, you'll feel drowsy, grumpy, and not awake for hours. Babies work the same as we do, so take some time to write down how your baby wakes up. Do you wake your baby from a deep sleep when you need to go to an appointment? Or does your baby wake naturally and is happy? This can help give you clues to your baby's sleep stages and cycle length.

Why does light or dark matter for sleep?

I'm going to get a bit scienc-y here. Light and dark matter for sleep because the circadian biological clock is controlled by a part of the brain called the suprachiasmatic nucleus (SCN), a group of cells in the hypothalamus that respond to light and dark signals. From the optic nerve of the eye, light travels to the SCN, signaling the internal clock that it is time to be awake. The SCN signals to other parts of the brain that control hormones, body temperature, and other functions that play a role in making us feel sleepy or awake.

Light exposure signals the body to wake up by raising our body temperature and producing hormones, like cortisol, to get our bodies moving. The opposite happens with darkness. Lack of light will induce melatonin production to get the body ready for sleep.

We need light to help wake up our bodies and the darkness to signal that it's time to sleep. Have you ever felt sleepier during the winter? This is because there's more darkness signaling your body that it's time for rest. The opposite happens during the summer when we get more sunlight. The light signals to the brain that we aren't sleepy.

· · · · · SLEEP TASK · · · · ·

Write down how your baby woke up today. Did you notice any of their sleep stages? How long were their sleep cycles (stages 1 – REM together)?

Why is sleep important?

This section isn't made to stress you out but rather to inform you about the importance of sleep. It's important to prioritize sleep for both you and your child because it is our most valuable activity. More important than we tend to give it credit, especially for ourselves as parents. But keep in mind that babies go through phases where they may sleep less at certain points and that's totally normal too.

Sleep is critical for babies because growth hormone is secreted into the body during sleep. This is what makes your baby's brain and body grow! If they aren't getting enough sleep, then they aren't getting all of the hormones they need for growth and development, and during sleep is the only time your baby grows!

Sleep also helps develop memory, regulate emotions, stabilize hormones, such as blood sugar and digestive hormones. Best of all, sleep helps improve your baby's (and your) immune system. A well-rested child is energetic, happy, and playful, and rested energy is much different than over-tired energy.

Throughout the day, our brains produce *amyloid beta protein*. If our brains don't get enough rest, our brains can't flush out these proteins, leaving our brains full of toxins. Research shows that the quality of sleep we get as a child matters later in our life. If we don't get enough sleep, we'll feel fuzzy during the day because those leftover toxins didn't get flushed out. For babies (and for many adults too), that fuzzy feeling comes out as crankiness.

Keep track of your baby's total sleep time over the next few days.

Sleep tip for parents

If you find that you are also struggling with sleep, the first place to start is to reduce caffeine intake after 2:00 pm because, depending on how you metabolize caffeine, it can stay in your system for up to 8 – 10 hours. I know, caffeine is basically your lifeline when your child isn't sleeping, but switch to decaffeinated or caffeine-free coffee or drink a decaf or caffeine-free tea later in the day. The reason is because caffeine blocks adenosine (the sleep pressure hormone) from binding to its receptors and inducing that sleepy feeling, which is great during the day, but not so much at night when it can disrupt your ability to sleep.

Now that you know how sleep cycles work, understand why your baby wakes up in a sleep cycle, and the importance of sleep, let's move on to start putting together the sleep puzzle. We're going to talk about routines, naps, room environment, sleep props, and more in the next chapter!

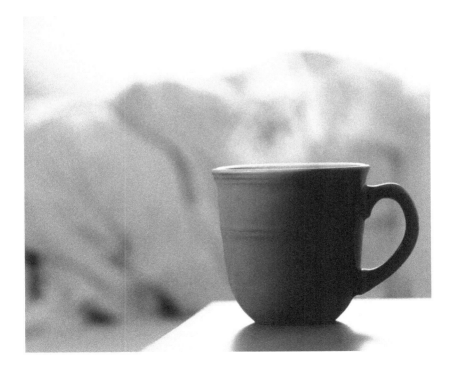

Happy sleep basics

First, we'll focus on setting up for sleep success. If you jump straight into sleep training, then you will have trouble because your child's body isn't ready for the adjustment.

Week 1

This section is perfect for any age group, as it helps set up the body for sleep. For babies under five months old, you will only be working on this stage because their sleep cycles will be changing at a rapid pace and you won't find a strong pattern to their days just yet.

While this section can be done within a week, take as much time as you need to get these steps in place. Some sections, however, you may be able to skip right over if it doesn't apply to you.

> ★ Remember, work through Week 1 before moving onto Weeks 3 & 4 in Chapter 5.

The first week I recommend that you work on these parts and allow your baby to ease into the new way of sleeping. I also advise that you write down a plan (there's space in the back of the book to write this down. You'll find this in the *Appendix*) on when and how you'll make these changes. This will help you stick to your plan and also keep you and anyone else caring for your child on the same page.

From this chapter, choose two to three items to work on each day of the week until you have covered this list:

- Your baby's wake window
- Timing of your baby's naps
- Sleep props – positive and negative sleep associations
- Room environment
- Nap and bedtime routines
- Sleeping phrase
- Consistency

Before you begin

Describe how sleep is right now for your family. Describe how the situation is affecting you and your family, and why you want to make changes. This is an important step because this will help you evaluate how sleep changes are going along the way.

Sleepy cues

When a baby starts getting closer to their awake window closing, they will often show signs to let you know when it's time to get ready for sleep. These signs can include:

- Red eyebrows
- Pulling ears
- Pulling hair
- Looking away
- Staring blankly
- Cranky
- Yawning
- Making jerky arm and leg movements
- Arching backwards
- Frowning or looking worried
- Sucking on fingers – this could be a good sign and might mean that your baby is trying to find ways to settle to sleep

For older babies you might also see some of these signs:

- Clumsiness, such as falling down more
- Clinginess, needing more attention, and wanting to be close
- Crying or general fussiness
- Becoming bored with toys
- Fussiness with food

Your child may have other signs, so be sure to notice what they do when their awake-window (see next sections) starts to close. These signs help you know when it's time to reduce stimulation and start getting your baby ready for sleep. By knowing these signs, you can help reduce over-tiredness and the possibility of your baby being harder to settle to sleep.

· · · · · **SLEEP TASK** · · · · ·

What are your child's sleepy cues?

Awake windows

An awake window is a period of time that your baby can stay awake happily. Awake time windows happen due to sleep pressure within the body and are an important aspect to know because if your baby stays awake longer than he should, his body is flooded with the stress hormones *cortisol and adrenaline* to help keep him awake. This then makes it even harder for babies to fall asleep. That's where understanding awake windows comes in. By knowing how long your baby can stay awake, you can beat the release of stress hormones and get your baby sleeping before he or she becomes overtired and flush out those sleep pressure hormones.

★ Remember that this is a *general* chart and your baby may have a slightly different awake window time.

You can keep track of your baby's awake window by tracking the time over several days from waking up to taking a nap. Be sure to watch their sleepy cues (rubbing eyes, pulling ears, red eyes, red eyebrows, blank stare, etc.) along with the time to pinpoint what their awake time window is for their age. Knowing this awake window will also allow for your child to develop a circadian rhythm, which is your baby's natural sleep and wake cycle.

Some babies will also do well with a gradual awake window. This means that they can handle more or less sleep as the day goes on. Use the *Sleep Log in the Appendix* (page 196) to keep track of what works best for your baby.

Age (months)	General awake window between naps	Daily sleep requirements	Number of naps	Wake if nap is longer than
Newborn	45 min – 1 hour	14 – 19 hours	3 – 5	3 hours
3 – 6	1.5 – 2 hours	13 – 16 hours	3 – 4	2 – 3 hours
6 – 13	2.5 – 3.5 hours	12 – 16 hours	2 – 3	2 – 2.5 hours
12 – 3 yrs	4 – 6 hours	11 – 14 hours	1	2 hours

Take down your baby's awake times for three to five days.

By using the chart for your baby's age and average awake times, you can figure out your baby's awake window.

My baby's awake window is:

Avoid over-tiredness!

An overtired baby will have a harder time sleeping and sleep for shorter periods of time. When their body is flooded with stress hormones, it makes it even harder for them to fall asleep and stay asleep. Over-tiredness often looks like your baby has too much energy, they can act hyper, overly cranky, and hard to calm. Watch your child's awake window and sleepy cues to help avoid being overtired.

Use the simple reminder of Clocks and Cues to help avoid over-tiredness:

* ★ Clocks = watch your baby's awake time window
* ★ Cues = look for sleepy signs

FOR BABIES 0 – 5 MONTHS, use their awake window and watch for sleepy signs. A combination of clocks and cues will help you set the right sleep times for your baby. Just understand that you may get it wrong sometimes (and that's okay!) or there's something else going on for your child. It's a fine line at this age between sleep and hunger, as cues can look similar. It will also depend on your child's temperament (read more about temperament on page 92). Some babies will not show any sleepy signs or very few, and go from a happy baby to a big ball of crankiness in 30 seconds, while others show very clear signs for sleep.

FOR BABIES SIX MONTHS AND UP, use the clock (awake window) to time sleep more than sleepy cues. You'll still want to watch sleepy cues, but at this point it's important to start getting your child's body on a rhythm for sleep, as this will help set the stage for consistency for their body. Remember that an awake window can still fall 30 minutes or so on either side of their actual awake window and the types of activities you have done that day may change that awake window. For example, if you've been to the park and played all morning, your child may show signs of sleep earlier than if you had been at home having quiet play.

Room environment

Your baby's room plays an important role in sleep. To encourage the best sleep, an ideal room should:

- **BE DARK** – so dark, in fact, that you can barely see your own hand in front of your face! Use blackout curtains or double up your curtains to block out any light from outside. If you need to use a light at night, it's best to use a red or yellow tinted light.

- **BE COOL** – 17 to 20 degrees Celsius / 65 to 72 degrees Fahrenheit depending on the season. Our body temperature drops naturally at night, which helps set the stage for our bodies.

- **HAVE WHITE NOISE** – a dull sound that helps drown out any other noises. Use a sound machine or a fan. Fans can serve two purposes: they produce a dull sound and also keep the room cool. More about white noise on page 46.

- **HAVE A SLEEPING BUDDY** – once your baby can hold an object, give them a blanket or stuffed animal (I love the combo blanket with a stuffed animal head). Make sure to put this next to your baby every time he sleeps (naps and nights), but don't use this as a toy. At first, the sleeping buddy should only be associated with sleep! Once your child associates this with sleep, then they can use it during the day as well.

If some of this sounds strange, remember that your baby came from inside the womb where it was dark, the perfect temperature, and had a constant whooshing sound. Re-make your baby's room to be as womb-like as possible and you'll have more success with sleep. This theory even applies to adults! If you have trouble sleeping, try out this room environment.

What's all the hype about white noise?

I'll use the term white noise here and throughout the book, but know that there are other frequencies as well that can be helpful. Noises can be described in various colors depending on the type of frequency they have. For example, light waterfalls can be described as pink noise and heavy waves can be described as brown noise.

White noise is mainly known for helping to block out household noise such as older siblings, city noise, or household noises. Some babies enjoy the sound of a dishwasher, vacuum cleaner, or hair dryer, which are all a type of white noise. For example, if you have a baby who needs a nap, but another child who no longer takes naps, white noise can help block out noises of siblings to help your baby sleep better.

Not only is white noise great for blocking out sounds, but some studies have also found that white noise can help babies and young children fall asleep more quickly. The research shows that many babies are able to fall asleep faster with a low, consistent noise in the background, as it helps calm the mind for sleep. White noise has also proven effective at helping inattentive children concentrate better in classrooms.

I'm personally a fan of pink noise and use it often when I work at my computer, such as when writing this book! Pink noise may have other sleep benefits too. Some studies suggest pink noise can actually reduce your brain wave activity. Your brain becomes less active during the initial stages of your sleep cycle. By using pink noise while falling asleep, it can decrease the time it takes to fall asleep, extend sleep duration, and improve overall sleep quality.

There are many white noise machines you can purchase, you can use a playlist, or use a fan. A former client of mine created a great playlist on Spotify called *Dr. Nighttime White Noise*. It's a combination of white, brown, and pink noise and I highly recommend checking it out!

Sleep props

A sleep prop is anything that assists your child to sleep. This is the most important aspect of helping your child sleep for longer stretches and also learn how to connect their sleep cycles from light sleep back to deep sleep. But this is also the most difficult aspect when you discuss child sleep. I'll cover stress levels soon (page 81), but know that learning how to sleep is no different than learning any other skill for your child. Sleeping well is a skill! And it's an important skill for your child's life and health.

Sleep props that may prevent sleep can include:
- Nursing/bottle
- Rocking
- Pacifier
- Mama or papa
- Co-sleeping

These are fine until ... no one is sleeping! Then these would be considered a negative sleep prop or sleep association. You'll know that what you are doing is disturbing your child's sleep rather than helping it when your child wakes up every hour or two at night and needs help going back to sleep.

Now, don't misunderstand that it's ok to help your baby a little bit with a prop to fall asleep, especially in the first four months. *Just be sure to reduce the time you use a prop to eventually let your baby do more of the falling asleep part by themselves!* Feeding to sleep is a common sleep association. It's one that is so cozy but unfortunately can also be the cause of many wakings as your child gets older. I generally have parents work away from feeding to sleep around four months old.

Positive sleep props
I often have parents ask me, "but isn't a sleeping buddy or bedtime routine a sleep prop?" Yes! There are also positive sleep props that we want to encourage because this develops positive signals to the brain and body that it's time to sleep.

Positive sleep props include:

- Good room environment (dark, white noise, cool)
- A consistent bedtime routine
- Sleeping buddy
- The same song or sleepy phrase each time they go to sleep
- Consistent awake time windows

There are other positive sleep props you can use. You'll know if you need to change the prop when your child starts depending on it to fall asleep again during the night.

★ Remember that everything you do is teaching your child and using healthy sleep props can save you and your family months of sleep deprivation.

What's the #1 mistake?

The #1 mistake parents make is not being consistent with the right props for long enough. Your baby will learn whatever you do on a consistent basis. If you try something new for two days and decide that it doesn't work, then you're right, it didn't work! The reason is that you didn't give it enough time to become "normal" for your child. Continue to use positive sleep props on a consistent basis and your child will understand the changes! Look for small changes to gain encouragement that they are catching on to the new way of going to sleep. *Small successes are big steps in the right direction for better sleep.*

· · · · · SLEEP TASK · · · · ·

Take a few minutes to write down your baby's sleep prop (if they have one) and how you'll reduce using the prop, if needed.

Your Sleeping phrases

A sleeping phrase is a verbal cue for your child to remind them that it's bedtime or time to sleep. It is a source of comfort for them to hear the same repetitive phrase and be reminded of what they need to do.

I recommend developing a sleeping phrase that is a short sentence or two, comforting, and relaxing.

Some examples would be:
– *Goodnight my little love, it's time for sleeping now. See you in the morning.*
– *It's time for sleep now, goodnight sweetie. I love you.*

I also recommend that you have a help sleeping phrase. You'll use this phrase to help guide your child to what they should be doing as they learn the new skill of falling asleep.

A helping sleeping phrase might be:
– *It's time to lay your head on your pillow and close your eyes because it's night-night time.*
– *Grab your teddy, lay your head down, and relax your body; it's sleepy-time.*

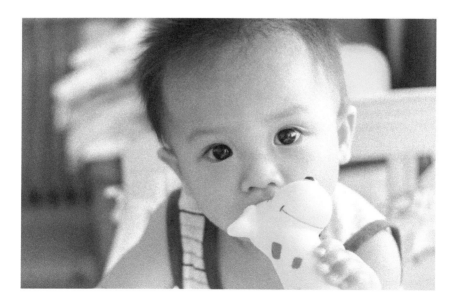

Take a few minutes to write your sleeping phrases to signal that it's time for sleep and also when they need a little guidance. It will be best if you say the same thing each time they go to sleep, but your partner or other caregiver can have a different sleeping phrase. It can also be in a different language, as well! Most importantly is that the same person says the same thing.

Routines

For the first four months of your baby's life, you will need to go with the flow when it comes to sleep times. Some babies will sleep more than others and that's totally normal! The only routines you'll have at this point include sleeping, eating, changing diapers, and repeating! There won't be too much in the form of routines regarding when your baby will sleep for the first several months.

There are a few things you can set in place early on. This includes setting up their room for sleep (dark, cool, quiet) and implementing simple and consistent sleep routines (for example, feed, song, sleep) to help develop these habits early on. You can begin simple routines as early as two months old. Once your child is around four months, they are usually ready for more routines and sleep guidance. Starting with these simple steps will help make this transition easier as your baby grows. Use the Clock and Cues guidance on page 44 for help setting sleeping times.

Why routines work

Some people love routines while others hate them. So, if you aren't a fan of routines, read this before you decide to use them or not. Also, remember that what you had in mind may not be what your child had in mind for having or not having routines.

Our bodies, adults and children alike, work on schedules and routines, and by using consistent routines, our brain has less stress on it and thus uses less energy. Our bodies and brains naturally do this to help us save energy, so no matter your opinion on routines, your brain will naturally develop them, be it good or bad.

Routines help our bodies set a circadian rhythm by using signals that help the brain develop an internal clock. These signals are termed a "zeitgeber," meaning "time giver" in German. While light is the main cue for our bodies, other signals such as when we eat, routines we have in our day, when we exercise, temperature, and even when we have social interactions also play a role. These can all be signals for the brain on how to set or reset our circadian rhythm.

Here are just a few of the benefits of routines:

- Put less stress on our brain
- Help our bodies to naturally react to a pattern called the sleep/wake cycles so the right hormones are released at the right times.
- Allow our bodies to digest food better because our body is used to eating at certain times; this is called metabolic memory.

These points are why it's important to have consistent routines during the day. Having these routines and habits will make your child naturally ready for sleep! I've experienced this myself, as well as with many of the families that I help. Simple routines can turn a cranky baby into a much calmer baby because they begin to understand what to expect next. It is the same as sitting down for food and putting a bib on or putting on their jacket and shoes before going outside. These patterns help them understand what one thing means and what will come next.

Day routine

It's a good idea to start simple routines early on because it's not only helpful for your baby, but also for you by not having to change how you go about your day as your baby grows! A consistent routine helps to develop a natural sleep/awake rhythm in your baby's body.

A simple day routine can look like this:
Wake • Eat • Play • (snack) • Sleep

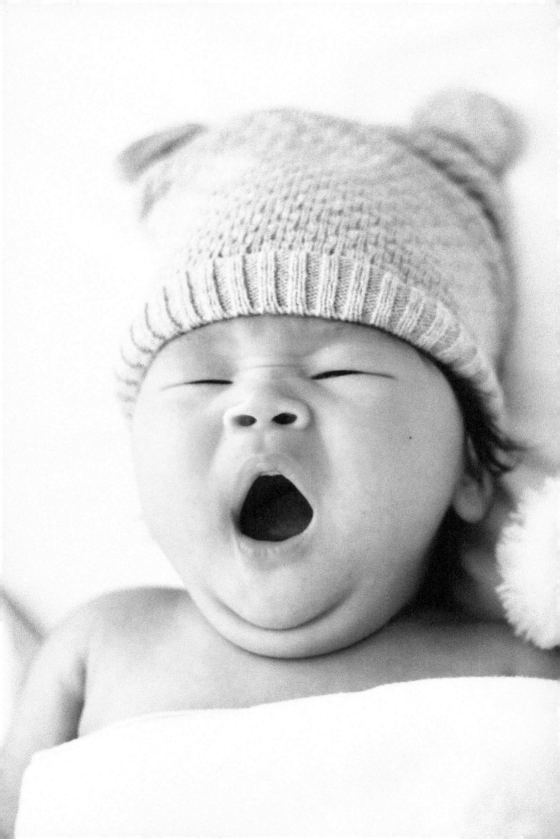

Nap routine

Establishing a nap routine is similar to setting up a daytime or bedtime routine. Your baby will begin to understand that this process means that they will sleep! Trust me, they are smart little kiddos and thrive on routines! Aim for the nap time routine to be short and sweet; between 10 to 20 minutes at the maximum. A nap time routine can look like this:

- Breastfeed, bottle feed, or light snack (but keep them awake during this time)
- PJ's (optional, but a good cue for sleep!)
- One calm book or calm song
- Bed

⭐ If you have trouble keeping your child awake during this feed, move the feeding 20 minutes earlier and also feed in a well-lit room. Then move to their room for quiet cuddles, songs, or books before bed.

Feeding is a common sleep association. It's one that is cozy but unfortunately can also be the cause of many wakings or short naps. If your child depends on being held or fed to sleep, check out page 46 for help on reducing this sleep prop.

> **CONSISTENCY!** This is the secret right here. Consistency is your best friend when it comes to establishing nap times and routines. Stick with it for two weeks before deciding if what you are doing is working or not! The most common mistake I see parents make is making too many changes or trying one technique for two days and deciding it doesn't work. Stick with it and be consistent.

Use *the sleep logs in the Appendix* to keep track of your routines, as well as to see changes that your baby makes with sleep.

· · · · · SLEEP TASK · · · · ·

Write down a daytime, nap, and bedtime routine for your child. Use the sleep logs in the Appendix to help track your routines and child's sleep.

Naps

As you now know, sleep is a 24-hour process and the timing, length, and quality of naps do matter, as we want naps to work with your child's body and help them to develop a natural sleep/awake rhythm (circadian rhythm). But let's be serious, even when all this is in place, naps can still be tricky!

The chart on page 42 is a reference for how many naps your baby will be taking depending on her age. Remember, these are guidelines and nothing is set in stone! One baby may nap better than another, take shorter naps, or not nap well. *Every baby is different and that is what makes general advice, well, general. This chart is a good place to start to get an idea of what naps might look like. Don't stress if your baby falls outside of these guidelines!*

Generally, the number of naps and when your baby transitions to fewer naps will look like this:

Newborn	4 or more naps
4 to 5 months	4 naps to 3 naps
6 to 7 months	3 naps to 2 naps
13 to 17 months	2 naps to 1 nap
24 months to 36 months	1 nap to 0 naps

"Help! My baby only naps for 30 minutes!"

Some babies will only take short naps more often throughout the day on a regular basis. If your child is happy and generally sleeping longer stretches at night, you might just have a short napper. You can try the advice below to see if this lengthens your baby's nap or if they really are just a short napper. Also, make sure their room is set up for sleep (page 45) and check if they are using any props to fall asleep (page 46). These can also cause short naps.

If your baby changes to only taking short naps, generally this can occur during a regression or because your child is sleep deprived. If they start taking short naps, try to go in around the time they usually wake and try to help them fall back to sleep. Work on this for a few days and see if that helps. Helping them might require using a sleep prop for a short time but this will be the first step to helping them sleep better.

If short naps are happening during a regression or milestone, then ride out the storm and hang in there as short naps are a common occurrence during these times.

Some babies will stop napping around 2 or 2 ½ years old. Try to keep a nap as long as possible but if your child is truly fighting a nap time or it is hard for her to go to sleep at bedtime, take out a nap and have some quiet time for rest during the day. Check for common regression times on page 76.

Can naps be too long?

Yes, naps can be too long and affect night time sleep! As you can see in the chart on page 42 there is a maximum length of time for naps and the reason is because we want to start getting your baby's body adjusted to being awake during the day and sleeping at night. Some babies will need help with making this adjustment and that's where waking them from daytime naps will come in handy.

Sleep really is a skill and babies will need time to learn this skill with your guidance. Their bodies are not born knowing that darkness means sleep. In fact, their bodies, like ours, need cues to let them know when to sleep and when to be awake. While some babies will make the adjustment in about two months, some babies need a little more guidance to make the switch; I know my baby did!

Keeping track of how long your baby naps can be important when figuring out night wakings. *Before eight weeks,* let your baby sleep as much as needed, but averaging daytime naps to be no longer than three hours. If towards the end of eight weeks your baby is awake more at night than during the day, now will be the time to start limiting day time naps.

As your child grows, it's recommended to limit the length of naps because we want their body to start getting used to sleeping in shorter stretches during the day when it's light outside and longer stretches at night when it's dark.

During some stages, your baby will take shorter naps and that's ok too. They will need a shorter awake window though, and be sure to watch their sleepy cues.

As a side note, once your child can stay awake for three to three and a half hours, keep in mind that their last nap time should not interfere with bedtime and to adjust their nap so they are awake long enough to be sleepy at bedtime. For example, wake your baby by 3:30 pm or 4:00 pm if they have a 7:00 pm bedtime. This will allow your child to have enough awake time before needing sleep again.

How to wake your baby from a nap

Waiting for the right time to wake your baby will be very helpful when limiting naps or even if you need to wake your baby at a certain time for an appointment. Here's where knowing the sleep stages will be very helpful! Remember that waking your baby during a deep sleep may cause them to be very sleepy and grumpy. If you plan to wake your baby, go in and see what stage of sleep he is in. If his body is very still and breathing is slow, he is in a deep sleep. If you can wait 10 – 15 minutes to allow him to complete the last dreaming sleep cycle, you will have a much happier baby! If you notice that they are dreaming (eyes moving, faster breath, or small movements), stay quiet, but go ahead and open the curtains a little to let some light in. Once they complete this sleep stage, they will wake up naturally. If your baby doesn't wake up naturally from the light, go ahead and wake them up.

Napping on-the-go

Staying at home for every nap can be impossible, but try to have naps at home as much as you can. It's good to go by the rule of 80/20. For 80% of the time, have naps at home. For the other 20%, you can be out and about. *If your child depends on sleeping in a stroller or a car, begin reducing the amount of time to 50/50. Nap 50% at home and 50% on-the-go.*

Why is napping on the go not recommended, you wonder? Because on-the-go sleep isn't as restorative for some children. For some children, their brain is never fully "off" while sleeping in a noisy environment or moving. Think about how you sleep in a car or a plane, for example. You are always aware of what's going on around you and although you sleep, you aren't being fully restored. Plus, napping on-the-go can become a sleep prop for your child and they come to depend on that to sleep.

If you need to be out instead of at home, develop a consistent routine or time that you are out so that your baby begins to understand this process. Last, maybe being out doesn't affect your child's sleep. Some children nap completely fine in a stroller! You'll know if this becomes a sleep prop if they depend on moving to get to sleep.

Reducing naps (and eliminating naps)

Once your child starts to struggle with falling asleep at nap times (i.e. playing instead of sleeping, having a hard time being put to sleep, or wide awake and happy) then it's time to think about changing their nap times and adjusting their awake time window.

When you reduce or eliminate nap times, keep in mind that your child will be sleepy or cranky towards the end of the day and might need to have bedtime 30 minutes earlier for about a week to adjust to less sleep during the day. Also, don't be surprised during this time if you start to have *more early morning wake ups*. Less sleep during the day causes more cortisol in the body, which in turn reduces the quality of sleep at night. Stay consistent and it will solve itself within a week or two.

When you stop nap time, the same applies as when you are reducing naps. Your child will be sleepy, cranky, might have more night wake ups, *and early mornings*. Again, be consistent! Put aside some time for quiet play or cuddle time so they have a small recharge during the day. Your child may also nap one day and then not need a nap the next day. Listen to what your child needs and make some adjustments while you take out naps from their day.

SLEEP TIP!
Use Clocks (awake windows) and Cues (sleep cues) to help avoid overtiredness and help set your baby's circadian rhythm (their sleep and wake cycle in their body).

Is your baby ready to drop a nap?

If you start seeing that your baby is struggling to take a nap, here are a few things to keep in mind. First, make sure that you have worked on your baby's awake window, have set up their room for sleep, and have a good nap time routine in place. If your baby still isn't sleeping well for their nap, consider if they are going through a developmental stage or regression time (page 76). When babies are learning a new skill, it can often interfere with sleep. Also, make sure your baby doesn't have any sleep props to help fall asleep, as these will often result in shorter naps. If those aren't causing short or no naps, here are a few cues that it might be time to drop a nap.

- Your baby doesn't seem tired at naptime and begins to have trouble falling asleep or it takes a very long time to fall asleep.
- Your baby begins to consistently have short naps (if longer naps were the norm before).
- The last nap is too close to bedtime and there isn't enough awake time.
- Your baby starts to wake earlier than before (especially if this wasn't an issue before).
- Your baby starts to wake more during the night.
- Your baby skips a nap here and there.

If your baby starts showing some of these signs and is within the age range of dropping a nap (page 58), then it's probably time to adjust nap times!

Three options

that I find work best when dropping a nap time

1 The first is to let it happen naturally. On some days your baby may take a nap and on other days they may not. This works well for easy-going temperament babies and also easy-going parents. This option can take around a month to adjust to the new nap times. You can read more about temperament on page 95.

2 Option two is to keep your baby awake by 15 to 30 minutes longer to help adjust to the change. Keep her awake with extra play, daylight, or a snack. Limit anything that can trigger sleepiness, such as breast or bottle feeding, car rides, or stroller rides. This option helps your child to adjust to the new nap times, but remember that your baby may be a little cranky when stretching their awake time. This can take anywhere from a week to a month or more to get on to the new nap times. You may need to wake your baby from the afternoon nap and/or bedtime may be a little earlier to help adjust to the change.

3 Option three is to directly make the change to the new nap times. Similar to option two, you will keep them awake with extra play, daylight, or a snack. Limit anything that can trigger sleepiness, such as breast or bottle feeding, car rides, or stroller rides. Your child will adjust fairly quickly (quickly can mean anywhere between three days to two weeks to make the change) but may be crankier while making this change. Bedtime may be a little earlier to help adjust to the change.

Remember, any change is like a mini jet lag and your baby's body needs time to adjust, which can take up to two weeks.

Setting up bedtime

Setting the right bedtime for your child's age will help her body develop a natural sleep and awake rhythm (circadian rhythm). An important aspect to this is having an early bedtime because this will allow your child to get the right amount of hours of sleep at night. *Don't be fooled into thinking that an overtired child will sleep more and longer, in fact the opposite happens!*

The other reason an early bedtime matters is because our sleep cycles change throughout the night. Not only does our body go through these stages, but take a look at when deep sleep stages appear versus lighter sleep and REM.

Deep sleep tends to happen earlier in the night and then our bodies switch over to REM and lighter sleep in the second part of the night. It's important to give your child the time in the first part of the night to get her deep sleep time.

Eliminate screen time

Screens include televisions, phones, tablets, and e-readers and if watching a screen is part of your child's bedtime routine, take it out and replace it with a book! Any type of blue-light will delay the release or production of melatonin and make it that much harder to sleep. If watching a t.v. show is around bedtime, watch the television show before dinner to allow the release of melatonin (the sleep hormone) into the body at an appropriate time. Take note that even if the t.v. is on and your child isn't "watching" the screen, they're still getting the blue light and resulting in heightened energy. Turn off all screens and have a calm atmosphere before bedtime.

I know many parents have started to use e-readers and if you do, minimize the effect of blue light for your child by using a nighttime setting and having the screen color as low as possible. You can also download a light altering software, like f.lux, to help reduce the blue light, or even buy blue light blocking glasses for your child to wear. These are also a great idea for you too! These aren't miracle cures, but they may help if you choose to use an e-reader.

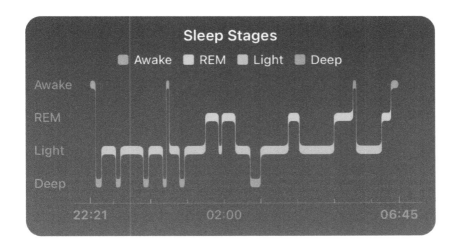

Sleep Stages

Awake   REM   Light   Deep

Awake
REM
Light
Deep

22:21   02:00   06:45

Bedtime routine

Along with setting up the right bedtime for your child's age, it's also important to have a bedtime routine. This routine should be around 30 to 40 minutes. If it's any longer, your child will not see the pattern as easily, so it's important to keep it consistent and short.

This routine, or zeitgeber (page 52), helps your child's body and brain transition into night time and also makes a connection that this process means sleep is soon.

An example of a night time routine looks like this:

- Bath (if giving that night) or wash cloth bath
- Pajamas
- Feeding
- Brush teeth
- One to two calm books or calm songs
- Bed

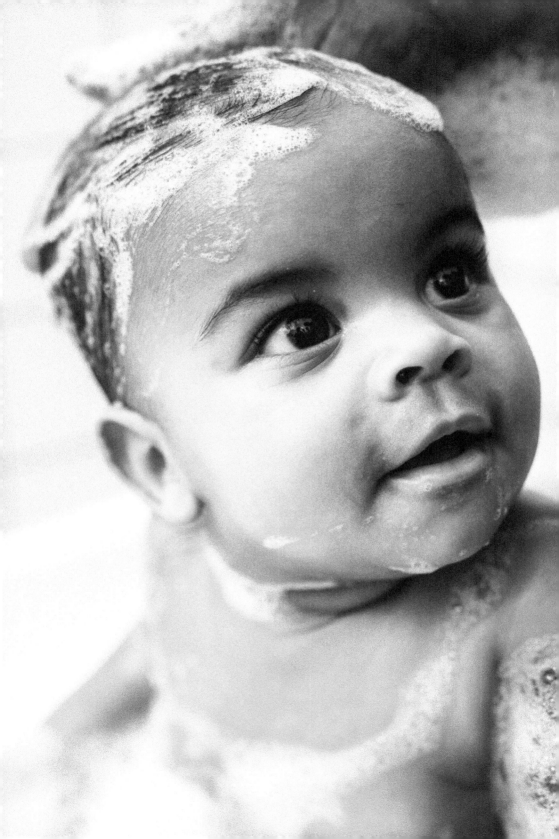

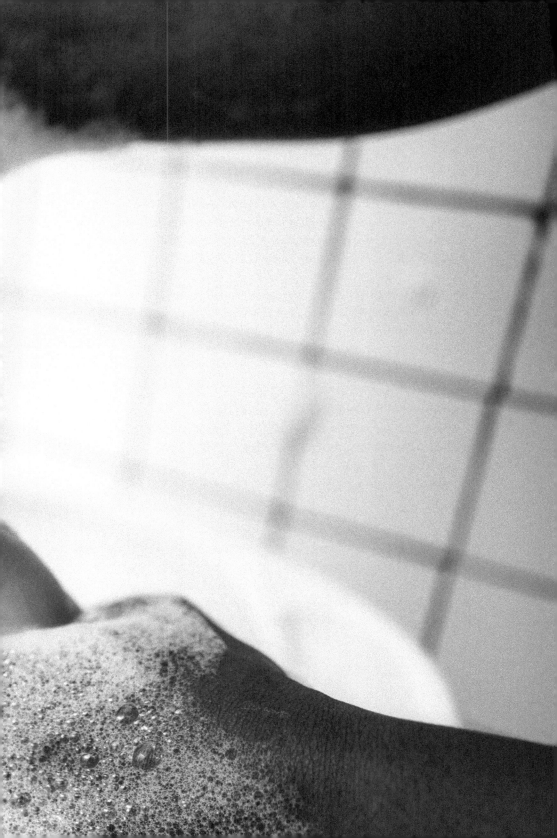

You can have other variations of a bedtime routine that work for your family, however, I recommend to keep feeding early in the routine so that your child doesn't develop a sleep prop for feeding to sleep. Feeding to sleep can be fine for the first two to three months, but after that, it's best to move feeding to earlier in the routine. You can have a simple bedtime routine as soon as you would like to help get you and your baby into this routine. If you find that your baby becomes too drowsy after putting pajamas on, then feed either before the bath or directly afterwards. The reason is because we don't want your baby taking a small rest and then having plenty of energy once she is put into her crib!

Remember to make the atmosphere calm and dim the lights to help your baby relax before sleep. Slowing down activity allows the brain and body to relax and prepare for sleep. So, keep in mind while doing the bedtime routine that everything should be calm after the bath.

CONSISTENCY, CONSISTENCY, CONSISTENCY!

I honestly can't emphasize how important having consistency is for your child to understand the bedtime routine process. Yes, it might be boring for you after a while, but this is for your child (and eventually you too!) to be able to enjoy bedtime!

Around 15 months, you can try using a bedtime routine chart to get your child excited about bedtime. You'll find a routine chart you can cut out to use with your child in the Appendix. Ask them what comes next in the routine and have them point to the next thing. You can also download the chart at www.HappySleepingBaby.com/extras.

• • • • • SLEEP TASK • • • • •

Take a few minutes to write your baby's bedtime routine. This will change as your baby grows and if you need to re-write your bedtime routine over the next couple of months, that's okay!

The last step … falling asleep

The last step to help your child fall asleep and learn how to tie together their sleeping cycles is to allow him some time and space to learn how to fall to sleep. This will be covered in Chapter 5 in more detail, but until you get there, this will help the process of falling asleep. This really is a skill that they must practice to be able to sleep happily at night. Just like any skill, your baby must practice it and he will learn!

"How do I help my child fall asleep without helping too much?"

Great question! What you want to do is reduce the amount of time you spend helping them to sleep. You can sing a calm song, rub their back, or say a simple sleepy phrase that lets them know it's time to sleep. Each night, slowly reduce the amount you help. It sounds easier than it is, I know. I've been there and I get it! *But continue reducing the time you help them and don't get stuck thinking they don't know how to do this!* Habits form easily and they will get used to what you are doing and make that their new sleeping prop.

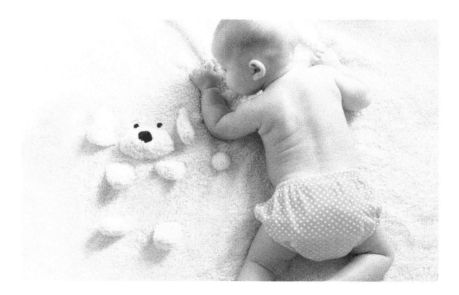

You can begin this stage by reducing your help in the following ways:

IF YOU are feeding your baby to sleep, feed them 20 minutes earlier and in a well lit room. Stop feeding once they start getting too sleepy and then hold or rock them to sleep. Do this for about one week and then move to the next stage.

IF YOU are rocking your baby to sleep, rock for a short period of time and then just hold still. This will help them get used to not moving to fall asleep. Do this for about one week and then move to the next stage.

IF YOU are holding, you'll work on putting your child down while they are slightly asleep. Stay close to them after you have laid them down and stay there for a few minutes. If your child is in a crib and you can't be too close, keep your hand on them for contact.

IF YOU are laying with your child, sit next to them and hold their hand or be close to them. Encourage them to use their sleeping buddy as much as possible.

The next stages of helping your child fall asleep are covered in Chapter 5.

We are always teaching our children to sleep. Anything that we do as parents on a regular basis teaches your child what to expect. Even rocking or feeding to sleep is teaching your child that this is how they fall asleep. They don't know that this will eventually change and this isn't how they will fall asleep forever! My philosophy is about teaching healthy habits and skills for both parents and children, so why not teach them healthy habits right from the beginning? You're giving them the gift of healthy sleep for life.

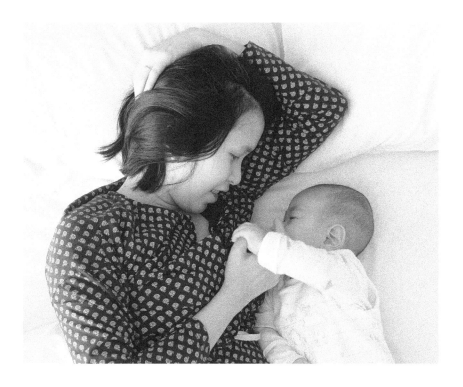

What about co-sleeping?

Co-sleeping is when you sleep with your child in the same bed. Some parents choose to go this route and others use it as a survival method just to get some sleep. I don't mind co-sleeping but it didn't work well for me since I'm a light sleeper. Any move my daughter made, I woke up. I would have loved to sleep alongside her but it ended up causing more issues than helping. In our case it was no-sleeping rather than co-sleeping!

If you decide to co-sleep, just know that your child may wake you up and it will seem like they haven't slept very well. Children move around A LOT. They wake up, sometimes talk, make noises, cry, or yell in their sleep. This is their brain processing all of the activities of their day and this is totally normal! I'm not against co-sleeping (we did quite often), but just know that if you choose to co-sleep, both you and your child's quality of sleep may be worse than if they are in their own sleeping space. This advice is also dependent on the child's age.

Now this may not apply to all children and families, therefore if you don't think co-sleeping is an issue for you or your child's sleep quality, then give all the other tips a try first to see what to improve on. If you are still struggling after working on many of the other sleep puzzle pieces, try putting your child in their own room for sleep.

Remember, a safe sleep recommendation is that a newborn should sleep *near* their parents bed up until six months to a year.

Setting up for sleep checklist

We've covered a lot of information so far and now is an opportunity to work on the sections that apply to your family. Again, this may take one week or more to set up. Here's a checklist to help you put together a plan for your family.

Awake window for your child's age (page 42)

Bedroom environment (page 45)

Your child's sleepy signs (page 41)

Chapter 4 for sample schedules by age (page 117)

Your day routines (page 53)

Sign language that we'll use (page 100)

Our nap time routine (page 56)

Our bedtime routine (page 64)

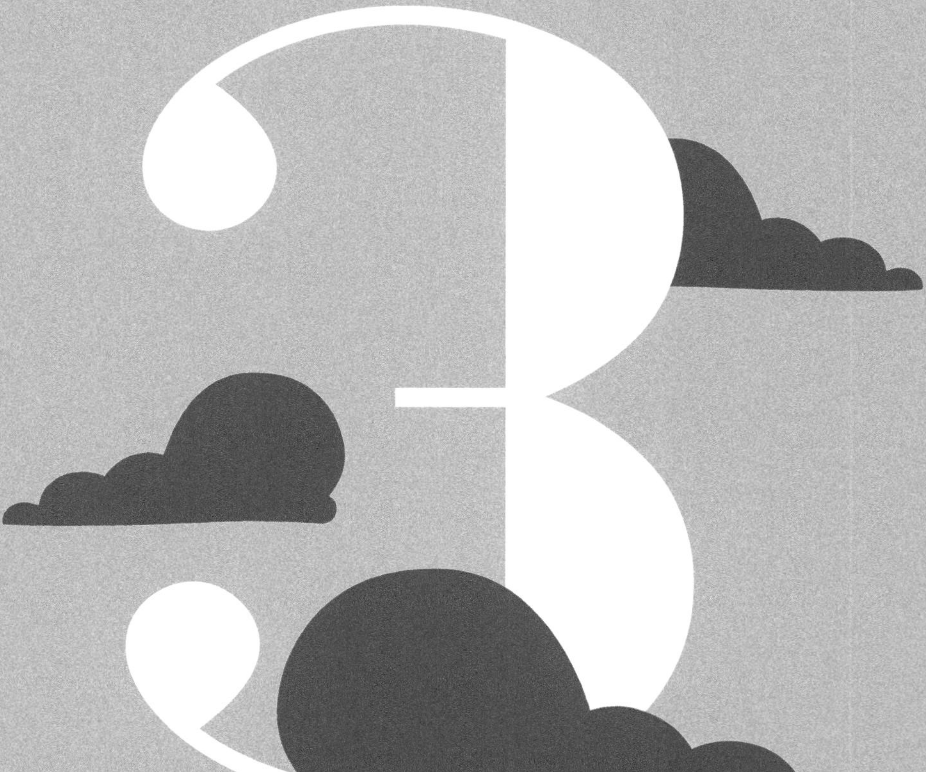
3

Factors that affect sleep

In this chapter, we go over information about regressions, development, stress, and so much more. Feel free to skip ahead to Chapter 4 to keep working on sleep and come back to this chapter at any point for more information.

What are regressions and milestones?

Regressions and milestones are times when all of a sudden you thought you had everything figured out and then it gets flipped upside down. The reason these happen is because your baby is constantly learning, developing, and growing, which tends to disrupt sleep. See these stages as a positive thing and that your child is developing just as she should!

These periods of time can last anywhere between two to six weeks. If you have sleep disruptions any longer than that, then look back at the sleep prop section on page 46 and if you began to use a prop to get back to sleep, then you'll have your answer. You can then start reducing the amount of time you are helping your child fall asleep (see page 167 or Chapter 5).

During these times you can expect your child to be a little crankier, want more attention, feed more or less, and have more sleep disruptions. Try to be as patient as possible during these times and don't hesitate to reach out and ask someone for a little extra help to keep your sanity!

Common sleep regression and milestone times

Sleep regressions may or may not coincide with milestones. I know, I know, it's not the clear answer you want as a tired parent! Sleep regressions are a bummer, there's no doubt about that. Often, the best you can do to get through them is to stay as consistent as possible with bedtime routines, bed and nap times, and limit your use of sleep props. Most likely you will need to help your child with sleep a bit more during these times. But the good news is that if you are as consistent as you can be, you will get through these phases before you know it. Another *positive fact is that when your child is going through a regression, it's confirmation they are developing normally!* You'll soon see new skills that your baby is working on!

Here are times you may start seeing your little one show signs of a regression:

- 6 weeks
- 3 to 4 months
- 6 months
- 8 to 10 months
- 12 months
- 15 to 18 months
- 24 months

Milestones show the same signs and are times of extreme learning leaps and that often come across as a period of crankiness, crying, clinginess, and sleep disruptions. Although milestones are tough for both you and your baby, again, try your best to think of these as a positive sign that your baby's development is on track. Your baby will have 10 major leaps within his first 20 months of life! That's a lot of development, so I can totally understand why they are cranky at times. Going through a leap is like waking up to a new world every month. When it's put like that, I'd be cranky too!

With that said, here are some of the major milestones your baby will hit and the stages at which you should be on the lookout. Keep in mind that these happen around these weeks, not exactly on the week.

MILESTONES:

Week 5	Developing senses
Week 8	Recognizing patterns
Week 12	Learning how to transition from one thing to the next
Week 19	Learning about events around them
Week 26	Relationships to objects and people
Week 37	Learning that objects fit into categories
Week 46	Learning about sequences
Week 55	Understanding more patterns and sequences
Week 64	Experimenting with the world of principles
Week 75	Learning about systems and consciousness

When your baby hits a milestone, it can be an incredibly exciting time, yet also really challenging. Your baby undergoes a lot of major changes during their first year and grows at an incredibly fast pace, so every month brings something new to look forward to with new skills.

One of the important things to remember when looking at milestones, however, is that every baby develops at his or her own pace. Of course, there is a (semi-flexible) timeline as to when certain things should happen, but for the most part, one milestone may happen earlier than expected, while another may happen a bit later. As such, the "window" for these milestones can be quite broad. So, if something doesn't happen when you're expecting it to, don't panic — try to enjoy the process and look forward to your baby's new skill(s)!

You'll find more information listed about these milestones by age within Chapter 4.

SLEEP TIP! The tell tale signs of a regression, milestone, or a leap in development is that your child is cranky, clingy, and crying more often.

I highly recommend *The Wonder Weeks* app or the book to track when to expect your baby's next milestone. Look at their website www.TheWonderWeeks.com for more information.

Along with other resources, I've used their recommendations for leaps throughout this book and while some kiddos will fall right in line with their charts, it's important to remember that some won't! Once again, this is based on general findings of their research and there can be some children who fall outside of those findings.

Nightmare or night terror?

Nightmares and night terrors are both scary and can cause sleep disturbances, but don't confuse the two terms for the same thing. Knowing some of the main differences can help you understand what's going on and discover possible steps you can take to improve sleep for your child.

Nightmares

Nightmares tend to be dreams with explicit, unsettling content, and occur most often during REM sleep when the brain is most prone to vivid dreaming. Because they happen during REM sleep, nightmares often occur later at night or early-morning hours when the brain reaches that part of the sleep cycle. Typically, someone who experiences a nightmare will awaken immediately with a pretty clear recall of the bad dream. Often, children will want to talk about the bad dream and have their parents reassure them that everything is okay.

Night terrors

Night terrors, on the other hand, tend to occur earlier in the night during deep sleep. A child experiencing a night terror may shout, sit upright in bed, sleepwalk, thrash around, have faster breathing, or appear scared for several minutes before relaxing back into sleep. Usually your child will only have a vague recall of the dream or won't remember anything at all. Although it can be distressing to witness, night terrors aren't harmful and chances are they won't even remember it in the morning. Night terrors can be alarming to witness, but they're not usually cause for concern or a sign of a deeper medical issue.

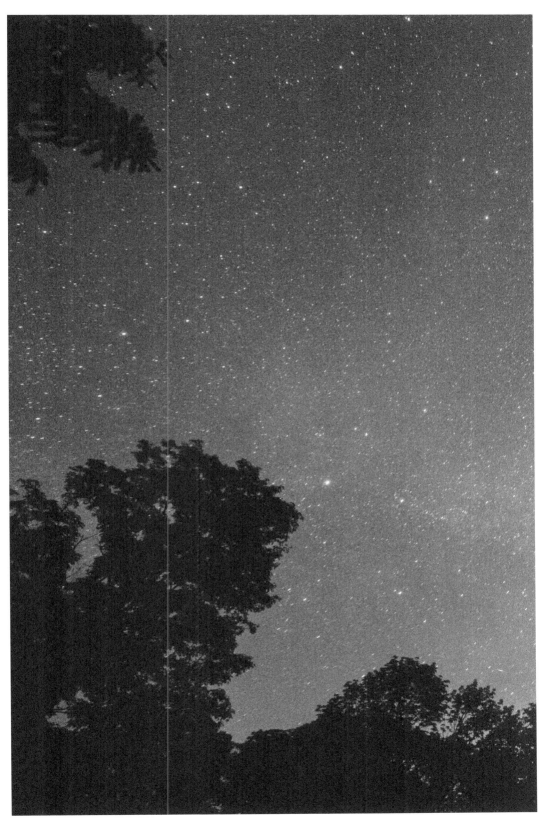

Night terrors are caused by over-arousal of the central nervous system (CNS) during sleep and tend to be more common in kids between the ages of four and 12 years old, but have been reported in babies as young as 18 months. They also seem to be a little more common among boys.

Night terrors have been noted in kids who are:
- Overtired, ill, or stressed
- Taking a new medicine
- Sleeping in a new environment or away from home
- Not getting enough sleep
- Having too much caffeine

It's best not to try to wake your child during a night terror. This usually doesn't work, and when the kids wake up, they are likely to be disoriented and confused, and may take longer to settle down and go back to sleep.

Night terrors are relatively rare — they happen in only 3% – 6% of children. Some kids may also inherit a tendency for night terrors; about 80% who have them have a family member who also had them or sleep-walking (a similar type of sleep disturbance).

While anyone can experience a nightmare or night terror, the latter is much more common in children. Night terrors typically go away on their own as a child gets older. Nightmares, meanwhile, can affect any age. A child might have one single night terror or several before they stop. Most of the time, night terrors simply disappear on their own as the nervous system matures.

There's no treatment for night terrors, but you can help prevent them. Try to:

- Reduce your child's exposure to stress
- Create a bedtime routine that's simple and relaxing
- Make sure your child gets enough rest
- Help your child from becoming overtired
- Don't let your child stay up too late

If your child has a night terror around the same time every night, you can try waking him or her up about 15 – 30 minutes before then to see if that helps prevent it.

Whether the concern is night terrors or nightmares, if frightening dreams are keeping you or your child awake at night for several nights (or weeks) in a row, consider talking with your doctor or your child's pediatrician. Sleep disruptions, whether you remember them or not, can negatively affect daytime energy levels, leading to a negative spiral of events. Discuss the situation with a medical expert to be sure your child – and you – get the good night's sleep you need.

Stress levels

The following doesn't only apply to sleep, but to a child's everyday life. I often get asked if making sleep changes will harm a baby, so I dug into stress levels and what's okay for a child to handle. If your baby has been fed to sleep for eight months of their life, changing that will cause some stress because it's a new skill they must learn, but it's nothing your baby can't handle. Sleep is a positive skill for your baby to learn and I think a few nights of learning better sleep skills is one of the best gifts a parent can give their child.

This information and research is from the Center on the Developing Child at Harvard University. They provide a lot of information for anyone to read and I encourage you to take a look at the reference section for their website if you'd like to learn more. https://developingchild.harvard.edu/

For a child's growth and development, it's important that they learn to cope with adversity. This is true for any situation, as their body must elicit some sort of physiological response as a mechanism to survive a "threat", which increases heart rate, blood pressure, or releases stress hormones like cortisol and epinephrine.

When a child's stress response is activated in an environment which is not necessarily a threat — for example, in an environment with adult support — the physiological effects that happen in the body are buffered and are returned to baseline levels, as there is no actual threat present. With this sort of response, however, the child's stress response system begins to develop. But if this stress response is drawn out over a lengthy period of time and there are no buffering relationships present, the systems may weaken, become damaged, and brain architecture changes, which may result in serious repercussions later in life. Research shows that long-term activation of the stress response system can cause impairments in learning, memory, and the ability to regulate specific stress responses.

But it's also important to remember that not all stress is bad. Stressful events can sometimes be beneficial depending on the body's ability to handle the stress and how long that response lasts. The response is also dependent on the duration, intensity, and timing of the event that causes the stress response, in addition to the context of the event. As a child's ability to cope with stressful events in their younger years has major implications for their physical and mental health in later years, understanding the consequences of stressful experiences helps parents determine more appropriate inventions to reduce the likelihood of later negative effects.

Keep in mind that the following three terms on the next page refer to the stress response in the body, not to the stressful event or experience itself.

Stress is a normal part of living and even babies can feel stress. Being born is a baby's first experience of stress. Yes, we want to protect our babies from stress, but some can have beneficial effects. We have *positive stress* every day, which is a normal and essential part of healthy development characterized by brief increases in heart rate and mild elevations in hormone levels. A positive stress example for an adult would be meeting a deadline at work or rushing to catch a bus. For babies, this could be having a wet diaper, feeling hungry, or meeting a new caregiver. The process goes like this: they are uncomfortable, they cry, we respond, they learn that we respond to their cry. This is a normal, positive encounter with stress. Positive stress actually helps us learn skills, too.

We experience *tolerable stress* when we go through any type of large change or have longer-lasting difficulties. These can include the loss of a loved one, a natural disaster, or a frightening injury. Tolerable stress activates the body's alert systems to a greater extent than positive stress. This stress is okay for children to handle as long as it's short-term, and the same applies to adults. The most important part is that we are there to help reduce this stress for them and guide them on how to handle it. Loving relationships will buffer the effect of tolerable stress.

Now *toxic stress* is what we want to avoid, if possible. Toxic stress is stress that is on-going and continues for months. This can be caused by neglect or by an accident, such as the loss of a parent and the child not having a constant caregiver, or a parent never responding to their baby's cries. An ongoing toxic stress response, or one that is triggered by several sources, can have a cumulative effect on a child's physical and mental health, both in the short- and long-term. The more adverse events experienced in childhood, the greater the risk is of having developmental delays and other health problems in the future.

Here's a breakdown of the types of stress responses and example situations. Keep in mind that these three terms refer to the stress response systems' effects on the body, not to the event or experience itself.

1 POSITIVE STRESS:

Every day, normal stress

Learning a skill

Telling you about hunger or a wet diaper

Getting an immunization shot

First day with a new caregiver

2 TOLERABLE STRESS:

Any type of big change

Loss of a loved one

A natural disaster

Frightening injury

3 TOXIC STRESS:

Neglect

On-going stress

NEVER answering your child's cries

On-going sleep deprivation

Why are you learning about stress? Because any change you make to your baby's "normal" routine will cause stress that falls in the positive or tolerable stress category. Sleep really is a skill, so sometimes we need to give our babies some space to learn the skill. And think about how your baby learns a skill during the day. They get a little frustrated, right? This frustration is no different during the day verses at night.

When it comes to sleep changes or training and stress, according to the Center on the Developing Child at Harvard University, "there is no evidence that, in a secure and stable home, allowing an infant to cry for 20 to 30 minutes while learning to sleep through the night will elicit a toxic stress response." While it's not easy to hear your baby cry, there's ample evidence that suggests that this isn't a bad thing when it comes to helping your child learn healthier sleeping habits.

HAPPY SLEEPING BABY

We can't handle our baby's stress for them; this is also a skill they learn. But we can help them learn how to handle their stress. Next, we'll cover how to help them handle their emotions, which in turn helps them with their stress.

Emotional regulation

(also known as handling emotions)

> Helping your child with their emotions will be a life-long task. Get ready for the ultimate test of your patience!

The second your baby is born she is learning how to express herself. For several months, the only way she knows how to do this is by crying. Emotional regulation is your baby learning what emotions are and how to handle them. Learning how to handle emotions and to self-soothe are very, very good skills for your baby to learn. I'll cover self-soothing tips in the next section, but first let's talk about what emotional regulation or self-soothing means.

First, this term doesn't mean that you will let your baby figure everything out by themselves and it doesn't have to mean letting them learn alone in a dark room. We need to take baby steps with them and be their guide. The learning process also doesn't need to begin at night, like many sleep training programs do. It's important to work on this skill during the day so that your baby can practice the skill at night.

Before we go further, I want to be clear that before four months of age, you need to attend to your baby's cries. I don't mean that they can never, ever cry, but you shouldn't leave your baby crying alone for a long amount of time. That's because they do not have the ability to regulate their emotions at this young age. You are their help as to how to calm their worries at this stage in their life. Don't feel guilty if you need to leave them to cry for a short time to use the bathroom or tend to an older child. This won't cause them harm!

A BIT OF A PUBLIC SERVICE MESSAGE: If you are so sleep deprived that it's becoming a danger to you and your baby, and you must leave them for a short time because you need a break from crying (for example, a colicky baby), please find someone to help you. Your baby will be fine for a short amount of time while you find help or take a quick breather. No one is a superhero and you will not be damaging your baby's long-term health. You are also important and need to be taken care of, too, in order to continue taking care of your baby.

Emotional regulation is one of the best skills that parents can work on with children because these skills are imperative for learning and development, but also to enable positive behaviour that allow them to make healthy choices. But keep in mind that children aren't born with these skills — they are born with the potential to develop them. Some children may need more support than others to develop these skills.

According to the Center on the Developing Child at Harvard University, the development of emotional regulation depends on three main brain functions:

1. **WORKING MEMORY** Controls ability to retain and manipulate specific information over a short time.
2. **MENTAL FLEXIBILITY** Helps to sustain or direct attention to different demands.
3. **SELF-CONTROL** Enables prioritization or ability to resist impulsive actions or responses.

Providing the support that children need to build the skill of handling their emotions at home, in early care and education programs, and in other settings they experience regularly is one of society's most important responsibilities. Environments that provide children with the groundwork and guidance to help them practice these skills before performing them alone is the optimal setting for learning. Parents and caregivers can help the development of a child's skills by establishing routines, modeling social behavior, and creating and maintaining supportive, reliable relationships. It is also important for children to exercise their developing skills through activities that encourage creative play and social connection, teach them how to cope with stress, involve daily exercise, and over time, provide opportunities for deciding their own actions with decreasing help from adults. Developing emotional regulation is key for normal child development.

The main takeaway from this section is that supportive, modeling, and consistent adult relationships are important to help build the skill of handling emotions for children.

Learning to self-soothe

Many people hear the term "self-soothe" and unfortunately probably think of letting a baby cry alone and not being able to attend to them at all. When in fact, from day one, your baby is trying to develop a skill called self-regulation or self-soothing. While babies may go through a process of learning what to do with less help when going to sleep, it doesn't mean your child learns self-soothing from this process alone. In fact, handling emotions can be worked on during the day *starting around three months old.* You can work on this by allowing your baby to fuss (not full on crying) for a short time (starting with 30 seconds to one minute and then increasing the time) before you rush in to help. For example, if your baby is playing on the floor and starts to get frustrated, give her some encouraging words such as, "you are doing great, mama/papa is right here." You can also give your baby encouraging words when you hear them wake up, such as, "I hear that you're awake, sweetie. I'll be there in just a second!" Then you'll wait 30 seconds to one minute and then go to them. This gives your child time to figure out what to do and how to change her focus. Now, this doesn't mean you'll do this if your child is crying; I would suggest you practice this when they are fussing or happy. If you feel this is silly to give your baby encouragement, think again!

Our children listen to our tone of voice for reassurance and our responses guide their emotions and reactions. Signs of self-soothing can also be seen in other ways such as:

- Use a pacifier or suck a thumb
- Hold a blanket or stuffed animal
- Sing or hum (even small babies can hum as they fall asleep)
- Wanting to be close or asking for a hug

Why is this important for sleep, you wonder? This is extremely important for sleep because a baby who can fuss for a short amount of time and starts learning how to settle themselves down during the day will begin learning how to do this at night, too. Most babies will fuss when they wake up after a full sleep cycle and try to resettle back to sleep. This is a healthy skill for them to have because it helps them sleep, develop their confidence, and begin understanding how to handle their emotions. According to research done by the Center on the Developing Child at Harvard University, a baby who begins to understand how to handle his or her emotions will carry this skill on into adulthood and handle emotions even better.

In an experiment by Stanford University, called The Marshmallow Test, children mainly around 4 and 5 years-old were shown a reward, in this case a marshmallow, and were told they could either eat the treat now or wait for the researcher to come back and they would receive two marshmallows. This experiment followed the children over 40 years and showed that children who were able to learn how to delay gratification (wait for the bigger reward and handle the emotions of having to wait) tended to have better life outcomes, as measured by SAT scores, educational attainment, body mass index (BMI), and other life measures. Of course, behavior (and life in general) is a lot more complex than that, so let's not think that one choice a four-year-old makes about a treat will determine the rest of his or her life, but it's an important point to think about and work on with your child about learning how to wait for a reward.

In a later study done by the University of Rochester, researchers decided to replicate the marshmallow experiment, but with an important twist. The twist was that the children would experience either a reliable or unreliable experience from the researcher first before they were left in the room alone with a reward. Just a few minutes of reliable or unreliable experiences were enough to push the actions of each child in one direction or another. This shows that other factors are at play, such as experiences and the environment that surrounded children.

The situation has also been adapted for adolescents and teens, and has also revealed that middle- and high-school students who can wait a week for a monetary reward earn higher grades, show less problem behaviour in school, and are less likely to use cigarettes, alcohol, and other drugs than their peers who choose not to wait. All of these studies show that children who are able to delay a reward and regulate their emotions show a better ability to do this into adulthood.

But wait, my baby is just a baby, you say! Yes, I know and I'm explaining this because you can start *slowly* teaching this skill fairly early, around 3 to 4 months old. Remember, babies often fuss when they wake up after a full sleep cycle and can resettle back to sleep on their own. This is a healthy skill for them to have because it helps them sleep for longer stretches, develop their confidence, and begin understanding how to handle their emotions. This is extremely important for sleep because a baby who can fuss for a short amount of time and starts learning how to settle themselves down during the day will begin learning how to do this at night, too. Within each age section in the next chapter, you will learn what is age appropriate to help work on this skill.

For more information about handling emotions with toddlers, I highly recommend reading *How To Talk So Little Kids Will Listen: A Survival Guide to Life with Children Ages 2–7* by Joanna Faber and Julie King. It's a great resource for communication skills with kids during the tricky years!

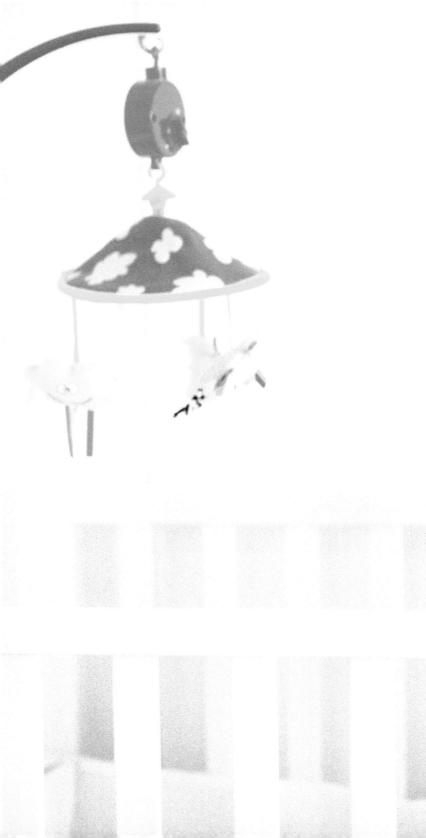

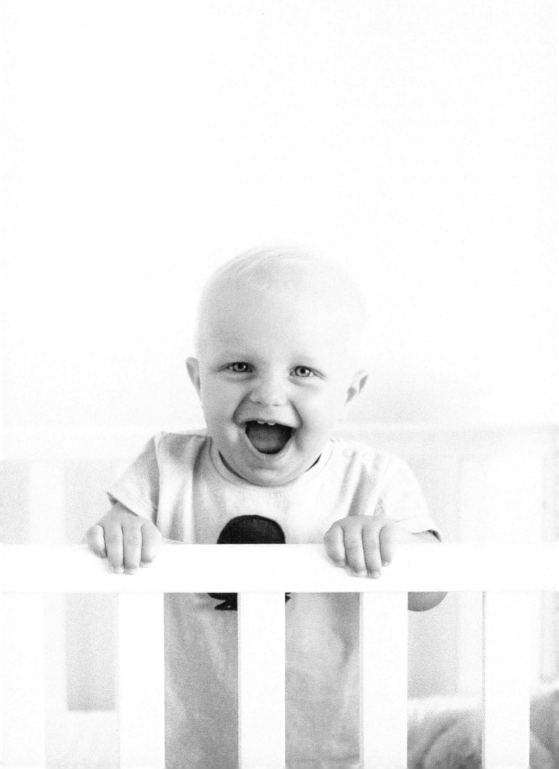

Consistency

Consistency creates success. Consistency also creates security for your child and builds trust, which is essential, just as the studies above showed. Your child will begin to understand what to expect during the day and when you begin their nap or bedtime routine. It still amazes me that when parents come to me for guidance and we begin with more consistency, their child begins to calm down. A once cranky baby becomes calmer and happier because he knows what to expect.

When you begin a new routine, be sure to give it some time. You might start seeing changes as early as three days, but if you don't, keep going! It can take up to two weeks depending on your child's personality, temperament, what you are changing, and if they are learning a skill or going through a milestone or regression period.

As I mentioned earlier on page 48, the #1 mistake that parents make is not being consistent with the right props for long enough. Your baby will learn whatever you do on a consistent basis. If you try something new for two days and decide that it doesn't work, then you're right, it didn't work! The reason it didn't work is because you didn't give it enough time to become "normal" for your child. When I work with adults I don't even expect them to change in three days! Continue to use positive sleep props on a consistent basis and your child will understand the changes!

Sensitivity & temperament

This is one of my favorite topics because this is what makes us all unique individuals. I started learning about sensitivity and temperament a long time ago because I found myself different then many people. I seemed more affected by everything around me and it bothered me that I couldn't just go with the flow of things like other people could. When I learned about the term "highly sensitive person" I found my answer. This led me to learn about these subjects and I feel I am a better parent because of what I've learned about myself. Let's dive in!

Sensitivity

Just like adults, babies have different sensitivities and temperaments. Some are laid back and happy most of the time; others can be prone to frequent tantrums. Some babies enjoy a peaceful environment; others feel more comfortable when there is noise around. You may not realize, but the type of temperament that your little one has can affect his sleep, as well as having an effect on any sleep training you provide.

When you are making changes to your child's sleep, he may respond easily and go with the flow or protest for a while about it. This is where knowing your child's sensitivity and temperament will help you when making changes and what to expect.

Understand that sensitivity refers to how your child *responds* to different environments and situations.

Dandelion baby

Now first off, if you have a dandelion baby, I'm not calling your child a weed! All I mean is that some babies are able to thrive no matter where they are and others need very specific conditions. Just like a dandelion, they can adapt and thrive no matter what kind of environment they are in, like this dandelion, for example. It's not an ideal place for water, probably gets extremely hot in the bricks, and the conditions are not ideal, but it's growing and thriving without any problem. Before becoming a parent I thought this is how all babies were. Oh, how wrong I was!

If you have an easy-going baby, the task of getting him to sleep through the night should be fairly simple. In fact, you may find that they do all of the work themselves. This type of baby can often self-soothe without too much of a problem. This means that if they do wake up in the night, they will usually fall asleep again in a few minutes.

If this sounds like your baby, you should simply stick to a regular routine each night so he gets to know that it's time to sleep. Self-soothers and easy-going babies do not usually carry on crying for too long, unless they need something. If the upset continues, it's a good idea to check if there is a problem.

Orchid baby

Now take an orchid. An orchid needs specific conditions that are just right to thrive. Not too much water, not too much sunlight, not too hot, not too cold, juuuuuuust right. If the conditions aren't good then the orchid doesn't thrive. I know because I had orchids living in Colorado and never had success with growing them, but in Sweden, they are like the easiest plant because the conditions to grow them are much better suited to what they need! If you have a child that needs very specific conditions, you know what I'm talking about. You'll need to be very aware of their awake windows, naps times, routines, and room environment for sleeping. Parenting will also take more energy with a sensitive child.

Every parent thinks their own child is special; even if their little one is difficult. However, some babies can be hard work; even if their parents will not admit it in public. If this sounds like your baby, the good news is that temperaments can change. Just because your baby is tantrum prone and attention seeking now does not mean she will be a difficult toddler or teen.

Orchid babies are easily disturbed and upset, and they want you to be there when they are. This results in frequent loud crying during the night. Orchid babies can go either way with sleep training. They either need a lot of help or helping too much actually disturbs them more. Here are some tips that you may find useful for an orchid baby:

- Stick to the same routine before bedtime
- Stick to the same sleep time
- Do not over stimulate your child with lots of new activities, especially in the couple of hours before the night time sleep starts
- Make sure the sleep environment is suited to your child. If they like a little sound while they sleep, provide it or use white noise
- As your baby gets older, try to distance yourself more; stay by the bedroom door instead of going up to the crib

Orchid babies will let you know if they are not happy and they are usually a bit loud about it. Be ready for this when making changes for sleep, or well, anything at all really!

If your child is a little of both

The fact is that many babies veer from being easy going to demanding at a moment's notice. There can be many reasons for this, such as:

- Changes to the home environment
- Changes to routine
- Eating different foods
- Upset in the home
- Milestones

Notice how your child is for the majority of the time and adapt your parenting to their temperament. Some children have a sensitivity level and they do not handle change or unrest very well. Others just love mischief and enjoy being playful in the middle of the night. These babies are often "signalers" at night. They wake up and they want you to know about it.

The best way to handle a signaler or a sensitive baby is to use a gradual approach to not answering their signals at night. You can start by popping your head into your baby's room to check on them, and then get them gradually used to you not coming straight away when they cry. If they wake up at night, you first wait only a minute or two. Then the next night you start increasing the time by another one to two minutes until you are up to ten minutes. If they just want to grab your attention and you do not provide it, they will often get bored and go back to sleep. However, all babies are different, so be prepared to be flexible. Some will be more persistent than others when it comes to this!

Temperament

Now, along with sensitivity, your child also has a personality temperament. This is generally how easy going or not your child is to situations and life. Keep in mind that these are general descriptions. Your child may be a combination of temperaments and will fit into more than one category. Your baby's personality also shapes how we are as parents.

Knowing and understanding your child's temperament can help her in different situations and also help you be a more understanding parent.

To recognize your child's temperament, you'll need to assess your child's activity level, how predictable they are (eating, sleeping, adapting to new situations), sensory threshold (how sensitive is your baby to lights or loud noises, dandelion or orchid), how loud or quiet they are, and their general mood. These clues will give you an idea as to their general temperament.

Here are some examples of common baby temperaments:

Unicorn baby

This is the easiest going baby E.V.E.R. This is a dandelion type of baby. On average, this baby is calm, easy to feed, easy to put to sleep, and doesn't fuss much. On occasion, she does become upset and is easily distracted, but calms down fairly easily. These parents pat themselves on the back and carry on with life as if not much has changed since their baby joined the family. Most likely you don't need this book!

By the book baby

This baby develops right on time. He experiences leaps and milestones precisely when he should, and all calming techniques work like a charm when he gets upset. This is a very predictable baby who can easily join along on a trip as long as food and sleep are taken care of for him! These parents know how to help calm and soothe him and he responds appropriately. They are able to set a schedule for the day based on his predictable body clock. This baby is more of a dandelion type.

Sensitive baby

This kiddo is sensitive to light, sound, and touch. This is generally a classic orchid type child. It doesn't take much for her to become uncomfortable and then tell everyone about it with wails! Everything must be just right and it's hard not being able to communicate needs with more than cries. She most likely will be sensitive to food textures and tastes. She will also need a dark, quiet room for sleeping, otherwise sounds and light will distract her. It is shown that sensitive babies have an overactive sympathetic nervous system that increases the experiences of touch and sound. Parents of sensitive babies know it because they will be standing on their left foot, feeding their baby with the spoon tilted at a 45° angle, and singing *Twinkle Twinkle Little Star* because that's how Baby Sara will eat her sweet potatoes.

Spirited baby

A spirited baby has a strong personality right from the beginning. Spirited babies are described as being ... more. More of everything. More intensity, personality, wants, high-energy, and intense reactions. Parents of spirited babies often feel worn out from the amount of energy their child has. As they get older, they are able to remember small details of events or point out little changes from before. I often recommend the book, *Raising Your Spirited Child* by Mary Sheedy Kurcinka, for parents with spirited children. Although sometimes exhausting, spirited children can offer parents a lesson in understanding people at a new level. When making changes to sleep for a spirited child, keep in mind that it's going to take a lot of perseverance from you as a parent. Consistency will be a very helpful tool for you along with setting loving boundaries.

> Time for a little self-reflection on your own temperament! Do you recognize any of the same traits in yourself?

By the time you are ready to make changes for your baby to sleep, you should have a good idea of their personality and how it will affect making sleep changes.

> Further reading suggestions from this section:
>
> *Raising Your Spirited Child* by Mary Sheedy Kurcinka
>
> *The Orchid and the Dandelion: Why Some Children Struggle and How All Can Thrive* by W. Thomas Boyce M.D.

Talk, talk, talk!!

I can't emphasize enough how important it is to talk about the changes you'll be doing with your child. They are part of the process and getting them involved with what's next for bedtime routine, reading a book, etc. will help them enjoy the process. This is also great for their development because the more words and interaction your child gets, the more they take in! Start asking your child what comes next in the bedtime routine to involve them in the process and also see that they are learning! If they can't talk yet, have them point to what to do next. *You can also print out the bedtime routine chart from HappySleepingBaby.com/extras or take it out from the back of the book. You can also use simple sign language to help communicate with your child (page 100).*

Development benefits of baby talk

The more you talk to your baby, the more sounds, tones, and language they learn, which ultimately plays a big role in their language development and conversational skills down the road. While it might not be helpful to have a full out adult conversation with your baby, getting into some 'baby talk' — that is the high pitched, playful, exaggerated talking — has been shown to grab infants attention.

Around 80% of an infant's brain develops during their first three years of life, which means it's important to make the most of that time. As the brain develops, synapses start to form, which allows them to think, learn, and process information. Talking to your baby helps to fire up the area of the brain that deals with language and helps to strengthen those mental connections.

Here are a few tips to help with baby talk:

- Talk often, even if it's close to bedtime
- Talk while you're changing diapers
- Sing as you hold your baby
- Get some alone time, as one-on-one conversation is more beneficial than in a group
- Don't interrupt or focus elsewhere when baby tries to talk back and look into your baby's eyes as they respond
- Give them a mix of baby talk and adult language

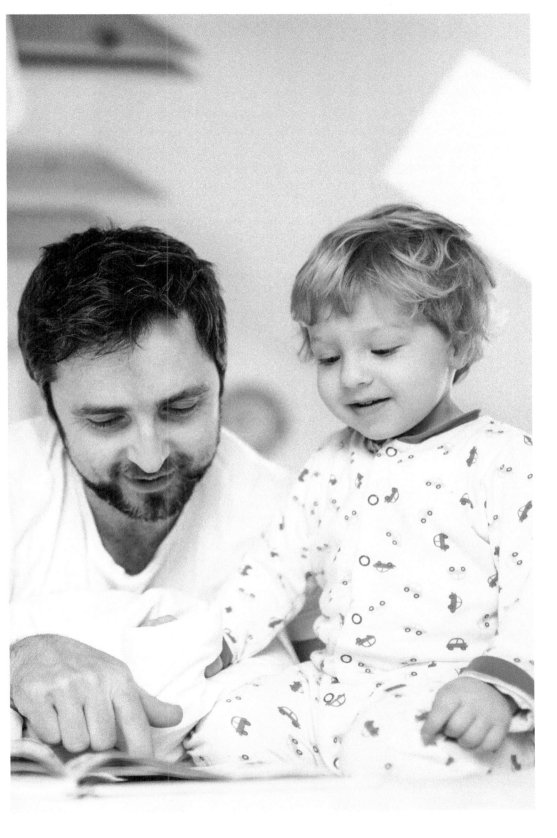

Talking with your baby fires up important synapses, which are connections the brain makes and needs to think, learn, and process information in the part of the brain that handles language. The more words your baby hears, the stronger those mental connections get. That process can strengthen your child's future language skills and overall ability to learn. When you talk to your baby and they happily coo, babble, and gurgle, you can encourage your baby to keep telling you more! It's fun and it's also crucial to their development. Your baby's brain is soaking up the sounds, tones, and language that she will use to say her first words. Infants and children who are spoken to know more words by age two than their peers and often tend to form stronger language and conversational skills than kids who don't. The only time you shouldn't talk is during the middle of the night wakings!

Using sign language

Another way to communicate with your child is by using simple sign language. Babies understand so much around them but they don't have the ability to talk even though they understand. Using sign language is a great way to help understand your child! It doesn't have to be complicated at all and you can start small.

Pick some simple, everyday signs that you can use with your child, such as:

- Food, eat, eating – pretend you are eating something
- Sleep, tired – lay your head on your hands and close your eyes
- Drink, thirsty – pretend you are drinking something

These little signs will go a long way in helping your child be understood! Begin by using the sign for "tired" or "sleep" or use your own by putting your head on your hands to show you are sleepy.

Development benefits of sign language

Sign language is a great addition to talking as your baby gets older. It is a great way to help with her brain development, as well as provide a bridge to the spoken word. It is believed that infants who use sign language also gain some psychological benefits, such as better confidence and self-esteem, and reduced bouts of anger or frustration from inability to communicate probably. Studies show that long-term, babies who engage in sign language at a young age tend to have a larger speaking vocabulary, an increased ability to form longer sentences, and are able to read earlier and have a larger reading vocabulary.

Additionally, teaching sign language to your baby may improve their visual and attention skills that are important for learning and social communication. If that's not enough, sign language is also a great way to bond with your baby. The interaction between a signing parent and baby creates a special bond that may not be as strong otherwise.

For examples of simple sign language you can start with visit: HappySleepingBaby.com/parent-resources

Pacifiers

Pacifiers can be a great help for soothing your baby, but once your baby is around four to five months old, it's time to transition to a different soothing method. One of the reasons is because pacifiers can cause night wakings and reduce the quality of sleep your child gets. This can result in a cycle of sleep deprivation. The brain is aware that the pacifier is gone once they wake up, which requires their body to fully wake up instead of a normal brief waking during their sleep cycle. Then this results in them needing help from you to either put the pacifier back in or help them back to sleep.

Not only do parents start eventually seeing better sleep once they stop using a pacifier, but many parents report that their child begins talking or making more sounds after they stop using the pacifier. Not using a pacifier also gives them a healthier way to calm themselves because they are able to know how to do this with a stuffed animal, blanket, or asking a parent or caregiver for comfort instead.

> When it's time to give up or reduce the pacifier, you are no longer using it during the daytime to help calm or soothe. When it's time to be done with the pacifier, it's time to be done! Otherwise, it will only confuse your child.

Reducing pacifier use

There will definitely be some upset and tears the older your child is since they have attached to the pacifier as a method of soothing. I advise choosing a date and making the change. Setting a date isn't for your child, but for you! It's much easier to say, "this is happening on this day" verses "I'll try today ..." and then give in later that day. Giving in will only make it harder for you and your child to make the change, as they will be more upset with uncertainty than the actual change.

No matter what age your child is, talk to your child before the change several times, and let them know that in "x amount" of days, things will change with the pacifier and that he will only be sleeping with his sleeping buddy. While your child won't understand days, it helps you plan and also get him ready for a change soon. It may seem like it can take weeks to get rid of the pacifier completely, but removal of it can actually be done in less than a week if you're diligent and serious about getting rid of it.

The easiest time to get rid of it is around four to six months old. The American Academy of Pediatrics recommends limiting or completely stopping the use of a pacifier around six months to reduce risk of ear infections, but there is no rule that says this is the age cap. Every parent knows that pacifiers can be helpful in stressful situations to calm their baby down. However, after nine months, attachment starts to happen and getting rid of it then can be a little more difficult, so prepare for a lot more fuss.

Pacifiers are so appealing to children because they help to relax their nervous system. Using other sensory activities may act as a good substitute to help wean them off use, such as:

- Bubble blowing
- Holding onto a stuffed toy
- Using a bottle with a straw (remove nipple to help sucking reflex)
- Towel rub after bath
- Squeezing toys
- Firm back rubs

Knowing your child's temperament will also help you choose which option will be right and also how your child will adjust to the change. For example, a by-the-book baby will most likely adjust rather easily with limited fuss, while a spirited baby will loudly let you know he doesn't like this new change.

Below are some options to help reduce or eliminate using a pacifier. For either option, you can use a different sleep prop, such as holding or rocking for a short period of time to help your child adjust. Just be sure to reduce the help over a few days or a week so that the new prop doesn't become a prop. These are not in a particular order; either option will work. Also, make sure your child's room environment, bedtime routine, nap schedule, and sleeping buddy are all in place first.

OPTION 1: Use it at nap time, but do not use it for night time sleep. Instead, give your child his sleeping buddy when he wants the pacifier. Help your child with some extra comfort to fall asleep.

While this sounds like the gentle solution, if your child doesn't start to understand the difference between naps and nights, it will not be a gentle solution and will cause more tears. Try this for one week and if you don't see even small changes, start with option 2.

OPTION 2: Stop using the pacifier at both nap time and nighttime and give your child the sleeping buddy when asking for the pacifier. Help your child with some extra comfort, such as rocking, back rubs, or holding for a few days to fall asleep. Be sure to reduce this help within one week, otherwise this "help" may become the next prop to work away from!

> No matter what option you choose, it will take some time (about four to seven days) for your child to adapt and if you are consistent with the option you choose, he will eventually adjust.
>
> If you don't think the pacifier is the sleep issue, make as many other changes (room environment, bedtime routine, nap schedule, sleeping buddy) as possible first. If you still have several wakings after one week, then the next step is to be finished with the pacifier.

Developmental tips to help sleep

Often a child will gain energy or act up at bedtime. This could be over-tiredness, but it could also be that they are excited or telling you that they need more attention. I've found that these simple tips can help a child fill up their needs during the day and reduce the need for attention at night. You're probably thinking, "more time for them, I don't even have time for myself!" but hear me out, this usually is shorter than you would expect. Just choose one each day or every other day and see what happens.

- **HAVE 20 MINUTES OF FOCUSED TIME** doing what your child wants to do. No phones, T.V., no distractions. Just play how they want to play!
- **WORDS OF ENCOURAGEMENT** and lots of talking about what you are doing. Talk about the bedtime routine, encourage them to help with the routine.
- **FOOD FUN** – baking together, helping with dinner, making a snack together.
- **CUDDLE TIME**

Why is this one-on-one time important?

Studies indicate that one of the key factors that helps build resilience in children is a sense of being connected to adults. Parenting in this way develops a warm, involved, and communicative parent-child relationship that builds trust. Spending time with and meeting them where they are at is crucial to your children's healthy development. Our children learn values from the adults they spend the most time with in both the day-to-day joys and struggles.

A study done by the American Academy of Pediatrics says that joy, shared communication, and interactions experienced by parents and children during play helps regulate the body's stress response. Studies also show that kids who receive one-on-one time do better in school, develop greater language skills, and have higher self-confidence.

One important thing to remember is that it's not about how much time you spend! It doesn't have to be an all day event! 10 to 20 minutes of one-on-one time is valuable. Your child will remember the overall relationship and sense of attachment they felt to you. They will remember the time you spent with them, having fun, and being there for them when they needed you. Of course, one-on-one time must fit into your family routine, structure, and children's age and developmental stage. The type of activity and time with them will change and evolve throughout their childhood.

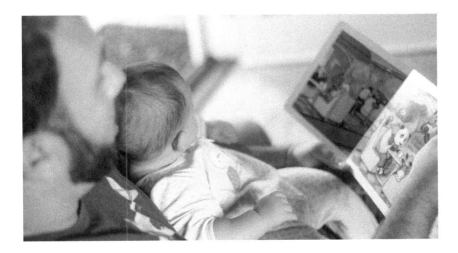

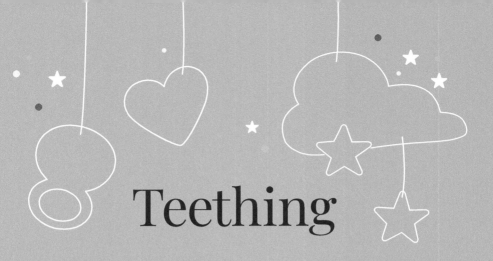

Teething

The verdict is still out on teething as to whether it affects sleep or not. Some parents swear that their child is in pain while other kiddos never show a single issue with teething. Basically, teething may or may not affect your child's sleep.

Teething typically begins when a baby is between six and eight months old, although some children don't have their first tooth until 12 to 14 months. The two bottom front teeth (lower incisors) usually come in first and next to grow in are usually the two top front teeth (upper

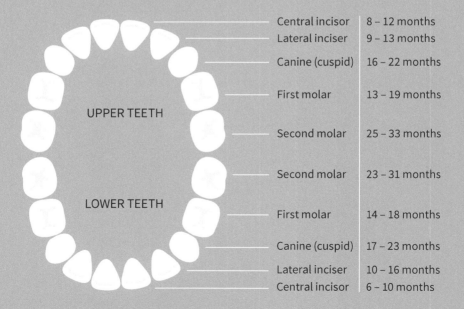

UPPER TEETH		
Central incisor	8 – 12 months
Lateral inciser	9 – 13 months
Canine (cuspid)	16 – 22 months
First molar	13 – 19 months
Second molar	25 – 33 months

LOWER TEETH		
Second molar	23 – 31 months
First molar	14 – 18 months
Canine (cuspid)	17 – 23 months
Lateral inciser	10 – 16 months
Central incisor	6 – 10 months

incisors). Then, the other incisors, lower and upper molars, canines, and finally the upper and lower second molars typically grow. All 20 baby teeth should be in place by the time a child is around two and a half years. Teething might be an issue if you notice that your baby seems uncomfortable and fussy during the day. Her gums may appear red, or swollen, or if you see a little tooth just below the surface of the gum, then your baby may be having some teething related pain and you can expect some disruption overnight. If you have had a fairly normal day and there is no tooth in sight, there is no reason to assume that teething is waking your baby. In other words – it's unlikely pain will pop up randomly in the middle of the night due to teething, and drool and mouthing of hands are not necessarily indicators of teething.

Teething affects babies differently, but here are a few things that can help with the discomfort and potential pain of teething – and to help everyone get more sleep:

- **USE A FIRM RUBBER TEETHING RING** for your child to chew on. Avoid liquid-filled teething rings, or any plastic objects that might break.
- **GENTLY RUB THE GUMS** with a cool, wet washcloth, or (until the teeth are right near the surface) a clean finger. You may place the wet washcloth in the freezer first, but wash it before using it again.
- **FEED YOUR CHILD COOL,** soft foods such as applesauce or yogurt (if your baby is eating solids).
- **USE A BOTTLE,** if it seems to help, but only fill it with water. Formula, milk, or juice can all cause tooth decay.
- **TOPICAL PAIN RELIEVERS** and medications that are rubbed on the gums are not necessary, or even useful, because they wash out of the baby's mouth within minutes.

Generally, teething pain will last a few days. If you notice that your child struggles with sleep, be sure to think about what sleep associations they have. Are they needing more help to fall asleep? This might be the culprit rather than teething if it continues on for more than a few days. Start tracking your baby's sleep and how they fall asleep to see what could be causing them to wake up and need help to fall asleep.

Your relationship after baby

Advice from a relationship expert

Most parents agree that there isn't a bigger source of joy and fulfillment than when they become parents. But rarely does an expecting mama or papa prepare for what is about to happen to their relationship with their spouse once the baby arrives. And yet, the biggest impact on your baby's well-being comes from you and your spouse, and the quality of your marriage.

Did anyone tell you what to expect in your relationship with your spouse once you became parents? Did anyone give you tools and strategies for how to survive and thrive together, not just as parents, but as lovers, as friends, as a happy couple, and as each other's biggest fans? If yes, then you are among the lucky few and I hope the tips here will inspire you further. If not, then you are like most of us who were surprised by how things change once there is a baby in the family, how our bodies change, our sex drive, our need for support, and for emotional intimacy.

So, let's look at what happens after a baby comes into your family:

- Your spouse and your relationship just went from #1 to #10 in the **priority list** and that is hard to accept. Nobody likes to see that they no longer matter as much, and for some spouses, it can be difficult to adjust to the new family structure and routines. We all have our **personal needs** and with a baby at home, these needs are often ignored. For a marriage to work well, you need to have your needs met and so does your partner. A sure sign your needs are not being met is if you find yourself or your partner swinging between angry and sad or positive with high energy and hopeless with no energy.

- **Your sleep** is messed up. The impact lack of sleep has on couples is less spoken about. It not only makes couples irritable and prone to arguments, but also decreases work performance, self-confidence, and overall health and well-being. Not to mention, the drive for romance and passion, or the ability to be patient with your spouse plummets. Some parents face a situation where their baby rarely sleeps and it becomes a sleep deprived nightmare. It's not only important for babies to sleep, but also important for couples to get proper sleep in order to have more strength to take care of themselves and their marriage, not just the baby.

- **Your privacy and personal space** are ... well ... non-existent. With babies and small kids around, going to the bathroom is a family event and taking a shower feels like a speed contest. That is a big stress factor! Especially for those of us who have strong needs for personal space and physical boundaries. Personal space and "me time" are more of a dream than a reality with some babies. And if you have no time for yourself, how can you talk about time with your partner for intimacy or passion? Some babies want to be carried for the first few weeks, which can be cute and cozy, but it can get to be very exhausting and it leaves little room or energy for intimacy with your spouse.

- **Peer pressure** becomes the cherry on top of the self-doubt cake. Families feel tremendous peer pressure, start to look at what others do, and see unrealistic social media images of parenthood. "Keeping up with the Joneses" or the "Kardashians" really helps the self-esteem, doesn't it? Yes, I'm joking here, but you get the point. The comparison trap is even more painful if you start to focus on what other babies the same age do and how your own baby compares, how others have lost the pregnancy weight, run a business, went back to work, etc ... This is a slippery slope and while these qualities can get you very far professionally, in parenthood they will only cause you stress and anxiety.

- **Social isolation.** Now that's a real bummer. This can really hit hard if you don't live close to family or friends, or maybe have friends with kids but they are not in the same baby phase. Parent groups and activities can offer some social contact, but choose who you hang out with and how much you do, as these groups can also add unneeded pressure. With my eldest, I was a very enthusiastic and ambitious first-time-mom, plus I was really lonely, sleep-deprived, and disappointed with how boring the baby phase was. So I filled up my daily schedule with baby massage, baby swim, mom groups, mummy-and-me training classes, post-natal yoga ... It only exhausted me further and the mom group I had only made me feel frustrated with how superficial the topics were and how nobody dared to speak about the real struggles in their relationships. If you find yourself in that situation, perhaps this can inspire you. With my second and third, I created my own group with women who were real, open to real talk, and supported each other. I only picked activities that helped me feel relaxed and valued, which made my maternity time more enjoyable and helped bring fresh energy into my relationship with my spouse.

- **Exhaustion.** "It's just a growth phase, it will pass!" If I hear this one more time, I might just check myself into a mental clinic! For most families, parenting is an endless string of tantrums, sleepless nights, chores, infections ... So how can anyone make time for dates, love, passion? Parenting is no joke and even if your baby sleeps well, it's tiring. You have a human to care for and keep alive!

- **Lack of intimacy.** Well, that should not come as a surprise by now, should it? Intimacy is about how free you feel to be yourself with your spouse and for your spouse to be free to be himself/herself. But with the lack of sleep, exhaustion, self-doubts, irritability, and endless chores, how does one even have the patience to just be with the other person, to listen without judgement or blame? And why does it even matter? Intimacy is like oxygen. Without it, any relationship suffocates ...

- **Low sex drive.** There are those lucky few who feel a boost in their sex drive after the baby arrives, but let's face it, most of you hardly find time to go to the loo and have no energy to even shower or shave your legs, so sex drive?! Hm ...

- **Romance** just went out of the window ... well, yeah. After an evening with tantrums, a dozen laundry loads, and several nights of bad sleep, who feels up for romance?

- **The past** rears its ugly head. Now that is a big one and certainly an issue that is rarely spoken of. When you become a parent, you are likely to start to relive your childhood and see certain childhood issues transfer themselves into your current relationship. Lack of unconditional love from childhood, abandonment, not being seen for who you really are, being pressured to behave well and achieve, arguments between parents, and "traditional mom-dad roles" suddenly make their way into the new parents' life. And … yes, there is more … Many parents start to reflect on what they lost becoming parents. Perhaps career opportunities, perhaps a great body and perfect physical shape, perhaps social life, intimacy, passion … the list goes on. The focus on what is missing may cloud the way you look at your spouse or how he/she looks at you and makes it hard to speak to each other with empathy and compassion.

- Mother/Father-Wife/Husband-Housewife/husband-Friend-Lover-Muse-Professional, perfectionist, high achiever or free spirit? The struggle to combine **the different roles** is real. And it takes time and patience to make all the pieces of this new phase in life fit well together.

- And to spice things up! **Arguments, resentment, and blame** come into play. It is hard to take back harsh words, insults, or hurt. And let's face it, raising kids and keeping up a home is hardly ever a 50 – 50 division, so at any time there is always someone who gives more. And with all the points above, this can lead to resentment and blame.

- **Money matters.** Money is often cited as the most common cause of stress in a marriage. You and your spouse may or may not have talked about how you want to handle your money before the baby arrives, but with the arrival of a baby, and especially as your baby grows, your attitude towards money and your financial goals might change.

So, with all these things in the mix, how do you create your "happily ever after becoming parents"?

Here are a few tried and tested tips:

Don't solve the blame, solve the problem!

Take responsibility to meet your needs, be open to receiving support from your spouse, and help your spouse meet his/her needs. Safety, variety and excitement, love, connection, personal or professional growth, contributing to a cause – whatever your needs are, be clear about them to yourself and your spouse, be specific about how you want to meet these needs, how you want to receive support, and ask your spouse to guide you clearly on how he/she wants their needs met.

They say Eleanor Roosevelt once said, "All the water in the world can't drown you unless it gets inside of you," so do not be defined by your current situation. Take responsibility to create an even better future for yourself, your baby, and your family.

Think and act as a team!

Divide and conquer, and if the other person drops the ball, pick it up without blame. Invest in each other – time, energy, money, love. My personal motto is "whatever works," so throw away all the traditional norms, others' expectations, and "the Joneses and Kardashians?" Flush them down the toilet! Do whatever works for you, your spouse, and your kids!

Keep the flame of romance and passion.

The key to that is intimacy, and the key to intimacy is vulnerability and emotional safety. Tap into compassion and empathy. Be kind to yourself, first and foremost. Ensure you feel well and ensure your needs are met. Only then can you be strong enough to be present, supportive, and kind to your spouse.

Set healthy boundaries for you as a couple.

I know you might feel like sending your biggest cooking pot on its way to my head as you read this, but bear with me here and keep an open mind, okay? We live in a society that is very child-centred. There is so much pressure to put your child first, but there is a BIG problem with that notion. If you sacrifice yourself, your partner, or your relationship in the process, your child will actually be the one to suffer. Safety aside, the best thing for a child is a happy home! So take good care of yourself and your spouse, talk about your boundaries, what you will and will not tolerate in your relationship, your priorities, and values and goals, including the financial aspects of these.

Praise your partner in public! And don't be afraid to apologize in public!
A compliment is 100 times more powerful if you say it in public. Lead by example. You do that easily for your child, so why not do it for your spouse, too?

Always align your parenting strategies.
This is another one where you might feel like throwing a pan in my direction, but again, "Do it now. Believe it later." So listen up! The agreement between parents is more important than what they agree on. Food, sweets, screen time, sleep time, discipline, learning – to your child it matters more that you agree than what you actually agree on. Research data on what food and routine is best for your child changes all the time, so don't get stuck on the latest research and don't immediately set your rules by that. Find out what you and your partner can agree on and then make that the rule. I always suggest my clients use the "rule of 3," or as they put it in Charmed, "the power of three, will set you free." Three rules for your child, that is all it takes. The rest is up for negotiations, which by the way, is a great way to teach your child good influence and negotiation skills. Your three rules will change as your child grows and their needs change. The key is to discuss these and agree on them in advance so you can speak one voice in front of your child and avoid arguments on the important matters. And if you happen to disagree or argue in front of your child, that is okay. Make up in front of your child. This will help your child understand that an argument or disagreement is not the end of the love.

Dare to be vulnerable and ask for help.
Whatever it is that you are struggling with right now, find the strength and courage in you to ask for help. There is no reward in suffering and

those of us who are strong and high-achievers often have the most diffi-culty asking for help and showing vulnerability. But there is huge power in vulnerability. Tap into it and ask for help. If you do not get it, ask again or ask someone else. Think of it this way. If your child was in your situation and needed help, what would you want your child to do? Suffer through it alone or get help?

I hope these tips can help you and your partner develop a healthy relationship as you create a family together!

With wishes for you to live, laugh, love and parent with inner power, passion and purpose.
~Polya

POLYA ROSIN helps couples create healthy relationships for a happy life. She is a certified coach and scientist with over 11 years experi-ence in health and well-being. She is a mama of three kids, an expat since the age of 18, has a multicultural bonus family, and is a strong advocate for a passionate life and happy families. Contact Polya at polya@polyarosin.com or visit https://polyarosin.com/ for support and to find out how you can apply these tips to your specific situa-tion and create your "happily ever after" once the baby arrives.

Sometimes it's difficult to fall back asleep

When you're woken in the middle of the night, it can be difficult to get back to sleep. Hormones have helped you wake up and it takes time to get back into that calm, sleep state. If you find you struggle with this, here are a few tips to help you:

1 **AVOID LIGHTS** No matter the duration of exposure, blue light signals to the brain that it's day time and it's time to be awake, thus melatonin production slows. To fall asleep and stay asleep, the body needs to be producing melatonin. In order to allow this to happen, avoid turning on bright lights when you wake up and avoid looking at any devices with a screen. If need be, invest in a salt lamp or red light bulbs, as red light doesn't cause changes to hormone secretion.

2 **PRACTICE DEEP BREATHING** If you're unable to fall asleep, try deep breathing. Focusing on your inhales and exhales can help to calm the mind and allow the body to fall back asleep. Work on filling the belly with air with long breaths in and out. While your belly doesn't actually fill with air, this allows your lungs to expand and fill with air.

3 **KEEP YOUR BEDROOM TEMPERATURE COOL** Studies show that the ideal temperature for the bedroom is between 16 – 19 C or 60 – 67 F, depending on the time of year. As body temperature tends to drop during the night, you want to maintain this in order to get a restful and restorative sleep.

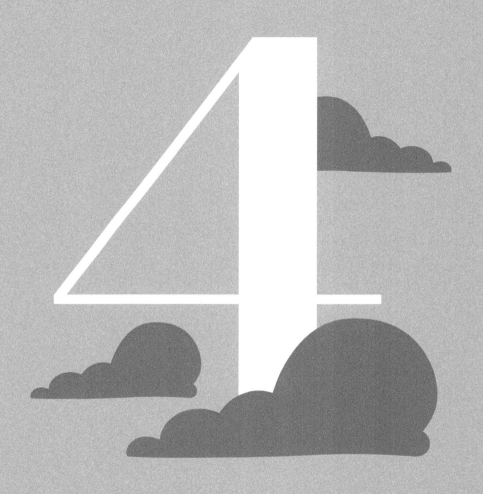

Schedules and development by age

Within this chapter you will learn about what to expect for your child's age. Learning about the changes your child is going through and what they need is key to helping you understand your child better. This chapter will be useful as your child grows and changes!

Within each section you'll find the following to help you navigate each stage in regards to sleep:

- What to expect and what you can work on during this time
- Awake window
- Day and night schedule and routines
- Sleep routines
- Sleep props and sleeping phrases
- Milestones and regressions
- Self-regulation practices

Keep in mind that you may see changes happen around the timeframe outlined and not exactly within the exact range. All babies develop at their own pace!

The first 8 weeks

Congratulations on such a wonderful and eventful time! One of the most important things to remember is to be kind to yourself because this is the biggest change in your life! This section is here to help adjust to your new life and enjoy your little one.

This stage is typically called the fourth trimester, which is the 12-week time period after your baby is out of the womb. It's a time of physical and emotional change as your baby adjusts to being outside the womb, and you adjust to your new life as a parent, either for the first time or with a new addition to the family.

Your baby is trying to adjust to life outside of the womb and Dr. Harvey Karp advises the following five S's to help babies adjust and help calm them.

1 SWADDLE

Swaddling recreates the snug comfortness inside the womb and is the cornerstone of calming. It decreases startling and increases sleep. Wrapped babies respond faster to the other 4 S's and stay soothed longer because their arms can't wriggle around. To swaddle correctly, wrap arms snug—straight at the side—but let the hips be loose and flexed. Use a large square blanket, but don't overheat, cover your baby's head or allow unraveling. *Note: Babies shouldn't be swaddled all day, just during fussing and sleep.*

Some cultures use body wraps or baby carries to help keep baby snug and close to them. This can also work instead of swaddling.

2 SIDE OR STOMACH POSITION

The back is the only safe position for sleeping, but it's the worst position for calming fussiness. This S can be activated by holding a baby on her side, on her stomach or over your shoulder. You'll see your baby mellow in no time.

3 SHUSH

Contrary to myth, babies don't need total silence to sleep. In the womb, the sound of the blood flow is a shush louder than a vacuum cleaner! But, not all white noise is created equal. White noise machines or louder fans work well to help calm a baby.

> I remember this one worked well for my daughter. We had to stand next to the kitchen fan vent or turn on a hair dryer! I also prefer brown noise to white noise but test to see what works best for your child. You can find many playlists on Spotify with brown, airplane, or white noise. One of my favorite playlists was created by a former client and it's called Dr. Nighttime White Noise.

4 SWING OR SWAY

Life in the womb is very jiggly. (Imagine your baby bopping around inside your belly when you jaunt down the stairs!) While slow rocking is fine for keeping quiet babies calm, you need to use fast, tiny motions to soothe a crying infant mid-squawk. To do this sway motion, always support the head/neck, keep your motions small; and move no more than 1 inch (2.5 cm) back and forth. I advise you to watch Dr. Karp's video on this at: https://www.youtube.com/watch?v=sB2Fw3MFlhk or Google the term "Dr. Karp sway". I also remember this one well because my daughter needed quite big jiggles to help calm down!

> For the safety of your infant, never, ever shake your baby in anger or frustration. Put your baby down in their crib and ask for help, if possible. If you don't have help, place your baby down in their crib (even if they are crying) and take a few breaths in a different room. No one is a super-human with a fussy baby.

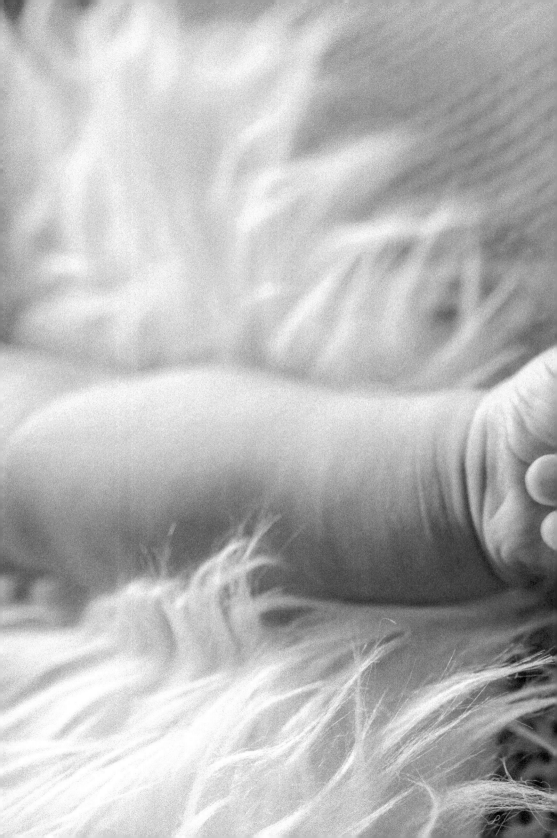

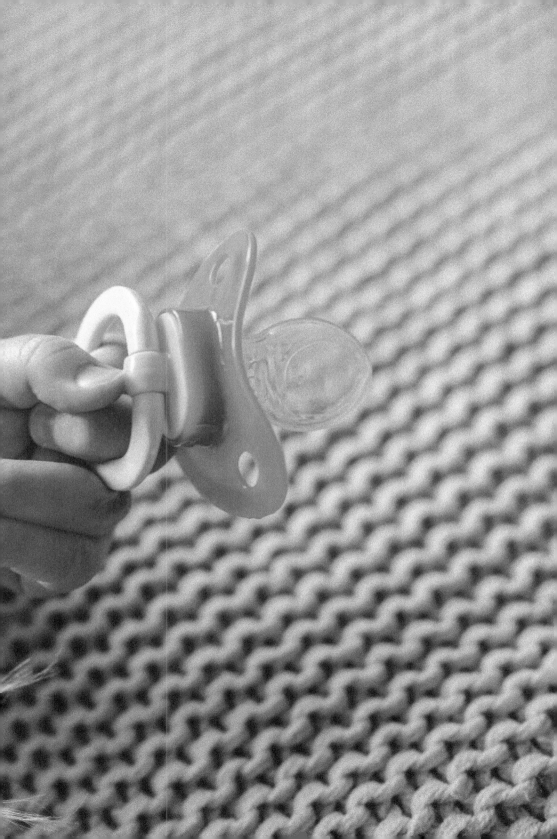

5 SUCK

Sucking is "the icing on the cake" of calming. Many fussy babies relax into a deep tranquility when they suck. Many newborns calm easier with a pacifier.

If your baby doesn't take to using a pacifier, don't push it too much. Some babies don't like pacifiers at all and prefer human contact. There's nothing wrong with your baby if they don't use a pacifier! Try using your finger or knuckle for your baby to suck on.

The 5 S's take PRACTICE to perfect

The 5 S's technique only works when done exactly right. The calming reflex is just like the knee reflex: hit one inch too high or low, and you'll get no response, but hit the knee exactly right and, presto! If your little one doesn't soothe with the S's, check out Dr. Karp's website at happiestbaby.com for more information to help calm your baby or, check with your doctor to make sure illness isn't preventing calming.

Other methods to help calm your baby include:

Skin to skin contact

Skin to skin contact is always encouraged in the moments after you give birth, but this type of contact should continue long after you have left the birthing room. Cuddling your newborn on bare skin is a great comfort to her. Your smell and the sound of your heartbeat is warm and familiar. This is also something your partner can do.

Feeding

Whether you are breastfeeding or bottle-feeding, if your baby is hungry, don't wait for a scheduled time to feed them. Combine feeding your baby with skin to skin contact to reinforce close contact and comfort.

Bath time

Having a warm bath is often a relaxing and comforting experience for newborns. Floating in the water is like being in the womb. It's also a great way for you to bond, talk, and sing to your baby. Yet, don't be surprised if your baby doesn't like bathing. It's totally normal too!

What does the fourth trimester mean for you?

For you, the fourth trimester is a time of great change. When your baby arrives, quite often the focus shifts to them and as a result, mamas often can overlook their own health and wellbeing.

Newborns take up lots of time. It's very easy for new parents to be overwhelmed in the first few weeks by the demands of feeding, lack of sleep, crying, and looking after a baby. Combined with the physical recovery after giving birth and the changes to their hormones, it's no wonder mamas can feel exhausted!

Don't be shy – ask for help

In some cultures, new parents spend the first few weeks totally focused on bonding and recovering with their newborn. While in other cultures, we take on this responsibility to be and do everything. Learn from mamas before you and ask for help!

If you have a partner, encourage him or her to assist and participate in parenting as much as possible. The two of you are in this together and there are lots of things you both can do to share the load.

You don't want a procession of people coming over, but a few family and friends can help by:

- Bringing meals
- Helping with household chores
- Looking after your other children (if this is not your first child)
- Looking after the baby while you rest

Accept help and don't be afraid to ask.

Eat good, nutritious food

You will need lots of energy in those first few months, so eating a variety of healthy foods will help give you the boost you need. Some light exercise will also help with your recovery and energy levels. But make sure to give your body time to heal and take it at your own pace.

Sleep or rest when you can

It might sound obvious, but you need to sleep. It's going to take a while for your baby to settle into a routine and even then, they will have you up at all hours of the night. If you can, try and sleep when your baby is sleeping, or ask your partner or a family member to look after your baby while you get some rest. Even if you don't sleep, take time to rest or do something you enjoy while your baby is sleeping.

When to see your doctor or midwife

Your body has been through a lot over the past 9 months. Your physical recovery will take time, but it's important to speak to your doctor or midwife if you have any of the following:

- Heavy bleeding or passing of clots
- High temperature or fever
- Offensive-smelling vaginal discharge
- A hard or painful lump in your breast
- An area around stitches that is red, hot, or oozing
- Pain, tenderness, or a warm area in your legs

Many women also experience the 'baby blues' in the first few days after giving birth, but if these feelings are not going away, it's important you see your doctor as soon as possible. Postnatal depression is nothing to be ashamed of, but you need to seek help.

What to expect and what you can work on during this time

The first 6 weeks will be filled with many feedings and naps. Newborns typically spend anywhere from 14 to 19 hours sleeping per day! It sounds like a lot, but sleep helps them grow and develop.

Here are a few things to keep in mind during this time:

- Although you will be feeding quite often, try to space out feeds every 1 1/2 to 2 hours. Spacing out feedings will help reduce gas and pressure on the stomach. But, feed your baby if you think he is hungry! In the beginning, it may feel as if you are feeding your baby constantly, and this is normal!
- Develop a plan between you and your partner on how to handle the multiple wake-ups at night.
- Let your baby sleep as much as needed!
- By the end of 6 weeks, test out if feedings can be every 2 to 3 hours in-between.
- Watch Clocks (awake time) & Cues for sleep. See page 44 for review.

Crying – is it colic?

Colic in itself is not a diagnosis but, rather, describes a range of behaviours that little babies will often display, such as crying for more than three hours a day, three or more days a week, and for more than three weeks. It is confusing and concerning to be told your baby "has colic" because it sounds like it is an illness or a condition that is abnormal. When the baby is given medication to treat symptoms of colic, it reinforces the idea that there is something wrong with the baby, when in fact, the *baby is going through a very normal developmental phase.* Crying for a couple of hours a day is normal; and in healthy, well and thriving babies, it is not uncommon. This doesn't make it any easier to handle, though, especially when parents try multiple strategies in an effort to soothe and calm their little one.

Dr. Ronald Barr, a developmental pediatrician who has likely done more studies on infant crying than anyone in the world, came up with the phrase the *Period of PURPLE Crying.* His idea was to explain this phase to parents of new babies so they would know it was normal and they would be encouraged that it would come to an end. The acronym is a meaningful and memorable way to describe what parents and their babies are going through.

The *Period of PURPLE Crying* begins at about 2 weeks of age and continues until about 3 – 4 months of age. There are other common characteristics of this phase, or period, which are better described by the acronym PURPLE. All babies go through this period. It is during this time that some babies can cry a lot and some far less, but they all go through it.

P – peak of crying
U – unexpected nature of the crying
R – resistant to soothing
P – pain-like expression on their face
L – long-lasting
E – evening or early afternoon when crying tends to peak

For some parents, having a guide helps them to understand that this period of crying tends to only be focused on the early months and is, in most cases, a completely normal manifestation of newborn behaviour and, although frustrating, is simply a phase in their child's development that will pass. Remember that this is only temporary and will come to an end. Do your best to use soothing methods or ask for help during this time. You can read more about PURPLE crying at purplecrying.info

Tummy Troubles

If your baby regularly arches his back, throws up often, or is uncomfortable in a seated position, it could indicate GI or reflux issues. It is common for babies to have some form of reflux as their food pipe (esophagus) connects the mouth to the stomach and is not fully developed until about a year old, but some babies have issues with this even though it's normal. This could interfere with your child's ability to calm down or feel comfortable. If you think this is an issue, avoid the positions your child is uncomfortable in; such as car seats or positions that put pressure on the stomach. Laying down flat may also cause uncomfortableness and notice if your baby is happier in an upright position.

Awake window

For the first months, watch your baby's awake window and limit awake time to 45 mins to 1 ½ hours to reduce overtiredness. You'll use Clocks (awake time) & Cues for sleep. See page 44 for review.

Day and night schedule and routines

For the first two to four months of your baby's life, you just need to go with the flow. The way your child sleeps will depend on basic needs, such as feeding and changing. But what you can do from early on is set up her room for sleep (dark, cool, quiet. See page 45) and begin simple and consistent sleep routines (feed, song, sleep. See page 52) to help develop these habits early on. Once your child is around four months-old, she is usually ready for more routines and sleep guidance but these simple steps will help make this transition easier.

Sleep routines

Your baby may not have a "bedtime" at the moment and may even go to bed for the night quite late while his body clock is adjusting to the 24-hour schedule to life outside of the womb.

Unlike adults, newborns do not have distinctive sleep stages until closer to four months. Rather, their sleep is categorized as active or quiet sleep. Active sleep is similar to REM and quiet sleep is equivalent to NREM. Quiet sleep characterized by slower, rhythmic breathing, less physical movement, and no eye movement. For the vast majority of their sleep, infants are in active sleep, which means awakening is quite frequent. Newborns spend approximately 50% of their sleep in an active sleep.

Sleep can be difficult for both parents and baby. Here are a few tips to help your newborn to adapt to a 24-hour cycle:

1 **INCORPORATE YOUR BABY INTO YOUR DAILY ROUTINE.** Your routine can help them adopt a 24-hour sleep cycle more rapidly than those who don't. When newborns are active at the same time as the parent, they're quicker to develop a more mature circadian rhythm.

2 **REDUCE NIGHTTIME STIMULATION.** When your baby awakes for a feeding in the middle of the night, try to reduce extra stimulation as much as possible. Do your best to avoid waking them up completely, which means minimizing interaction and keeping lights as dim as possible. A dim red or yellow light will help limit stimulation. Salt lamps are a great nighttime light when you need to change a diaper.

3 **ENSURE NATURAL LIGHT EXPOSURE.** Just like adults, natural light helps to normalize sleep patterns. While they may not do the job completely for a newborn, they do help. When exposed to more natural light during the day and complete darkness in the evening, sleep schedules can normalize quicker.

Sleep props and sleeping phrase

You cannot spoil a baby! During this stage you will be holding your baby, responding to their cries, and most likely helping them or feeding them to sleep. Do not stress over this during the first eight weeks of your baby's life.

Start using a simple sleeping phrase when your baby starts falling asleep. This can be as simple as, "Good night and sleep well my little love" or sing the same song as your baby starts falling asleep.

Milestones and regressions

There's a triple whammy around the six-week mark so don't be surprised if your baby starts to get fussy at this time. Most babies go through a growth spurt, developmental leap, and sleep regression at this stage.

Some common signs of this stage include:

- Increased fussiness and crying
- Increased night waking or shortened or missed naps
- Changes in appetite
- Extra clinginess

If you notice that your baby shows some of these signs, she is probably hitting this stage of development, which is great because it's happening right on time. It doesn't make it much easier to cope with, but hang in there! Around 6 weeks of age, most babies are growing out of their drowsy newborn state, and are starting to notice the world is quite overwhelming for them with so many sights, sounds and smells! Around this time they are hitting the development stage of developing senses, which is Leap 1 according to the Wonder Weeks.

MENTAL LEAP # 1: Leap 1 is all about development and happens around 5 weeks, sometimes 4. New sensations are coming at your baby from every direction, to which she will start to notice, but there is also a lot of internal development — from an organ and brain standpoint — happening at this stage. You may notice your baby being more alert as her senses are more sensitive than the first couple weeks after birth.

Self-regulation practice

There isn't any self-regulation practice at this age. You are your child's emotional guide and being close, available, and helpful is what is best for your baby. Babies at this age have very limited ability to self-regulate themselves without the help from a parent.

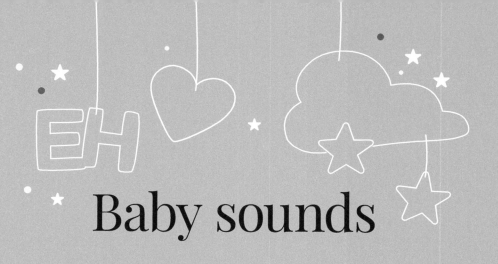

Baby sounds

Babies make a lot of sounds — there's no doubt about that. And while as parents we can learn to recognize some, sometimes we just don't have any idea what baby needs. Especially during the first few months when babies can't form actual words, they make what are called *sound reflexes*. While adults have reflexes such as sneezing and hiccups, babies tend to also have another set of 'reflexes' that indicate certain needs. Past the age of three months as your baby's vocalization matures, these sounds are eventually replaced with more elaborate babbling.

According to Dunstan Baby Language theory, there are five specific sound reflexes used by babies that parents should listen for. This helps parents detect and satisfy the baby's needs *before crying starts to escalate.*

The five sounds of babies

1 NEH (I'M HUNGRY)

The 'neh' sound is used to communicate hunger. It is produced when the sucking reflex is triggered and the tongue pushes up against the roof of the mouth. Other signs of a hungry baby are turning the head from side to side, sucking on fists, moving tongue in mouth, and licking lips.

2 OWH (I'M SLEEPY)

The 'owh' sound is used to communicate tiredness. It is produced in a similar manner to the sound of a yawn. An immediate response to this reflex will enable the baby to fall asleep much faster. Other signs of fatigue are eye rubbing and ear pulling.

3 EH (I NEED TO BE BURPED)

The 'eh' sound is used to communicate that your baby needs to be burped, and is produced when a large air bubble is trapped in the chest and the reflex is trying to release the air from the mouth. Other signs of needing to burp are fussing during feeding and squirming while laying down.

4 HEH (I'M EXPERIENCING PHYSICAL DISCOMFORT)

The 'heh' sound is used to communicate some sort of stress, discomfort, or that they need changing. It is a sound produced in response to a skin reflex (sweating, itchiness, etc.). As newborns lack the ability to regulate body temperature, they can easily become cold or overheated.

5 EAIRH (I HAVE GAS)

The 'eairh' sound is used to communicate either an upset stomach or gas, and is produced as a result of trapped air that cannot be released from the stomach or intestines. The sound often indicates that a bowel movement is occurring and can be confirmed if your baby bends their knees and brings legs towards the torso. Gas can also be identified by tension in the baby's body and face grimaces.

Recognizing the different cries a baby has can be difficult, but by actively listening to them, you can start to differentiate between each cry and the associated need. Each sound they make has an intention and a different meaning, so understanding each is important to providing the best care for your baby.

For more information about understanding your baby's sounds, visit dunstanbaby.com or HappySleepingBaby.com/Parent-resources.

2 to 3 months (8 – 12 weeks)

Your newborn is now a baby and becoming more aware of his surroundings. It's an exciting time filled with development!

What to expect and what you can work on during this time

Bed time might have been later before this time and now you can work on bringing bedtime earlier, anywhere from 6 – 8 pm.

You'll start watching for your baby's awake window and watch for their sleepy signs. A combination of clocks and cues will help you start setting up the right sleep times for your baby. Just understand that you may get it wrong sometimes (and that's okay!). There's a fine line between sleep and hunger cues at this age, which can tend to look the same. Some babies will not show any sleepy signs or minimal ones and go from a happy baby to a big ball of crankiness within 30 seconds. While others show very clear signs for sleep.

Use the simple reminder of Clocks and Cues (page 44) to help avoid overtiredness and start getting on more defined sleep times:

★ Clocks = watch their awake time window
★ Cues = look for sleepy signs

Awake window

Awake time will be around 1 to 2 ½ hours. You can read more about awake windows on page 42.

Day and night schedule and routines

Your days may still not have much structure but now you can start adjusting your days into 12-hour blocks of time.

Example of schedule and routines:

7:00 am	Wake-up, feeding, play time
8:30 am	Nap time (approx. 1 to 1 ½ hours)
11:30 am/12:00 pm	Nap time
3:00 pm	Nap time
5:00 pm	Short nap
7:00– 8:00 pm	Bedtime + nighttime feeds

If your baby is at a healthy weight for their age and size, you can increase day-time feeds to 3 to 4 hours in-between.

Does an early bed time really matter?

The answer is yes, it really does matter. And while it may not seem like it makes a huge difference to your baby's schedule, it does — even if it's just half an hour.

This is important to understand with respect to bed times because the non-REM to REM shift occurs at certain times during the night, regardless of the time you go to bed. Meaning, the later you go to bed, the less non-REM (deep) sleep you're getting, which can leave both adults and infants in a groggy state.

While this may not seem like a huge deal for baby's, as they sleep a significant amount, it eventually adds up. Putting your baby down too late or stretching your baby's awake period too long is a recipe for night wakings, restless sleep, and an early morning wake-up.

Sleep routines

If you haven't started yet, begin using a bedtime and nap routine at each time your baby sleeps. For example:

- PJ's and diaper
- Feeding (keeping baby awake)
- Book or song
- Bed

Sleep props and sleeping phrase

During this time you will want to work away from feeding to sleep if you have been. Feed your baby in a brighter room, talk to them, tickle their feet, or anything that helps keep them awake. It's now time to work away from associating feeding with sleep. If you still feed to sleep occasionally, it's not a problem, and if your child can sleep for four to five hours without waking, then it may not be something you need to work on right now. In my experience with working with families, it's best to work on this earlier than later as babies begin to associate feeding to sleep and it's a harder sleep association to stop later. If your baby has trouble with falling asleep in his crib, then after the feeding, place your baby on your shoulder or hold him to help him become sleepy before putting him down. You'll be using a differing prop (holding or rocking) if your baby has a hard time adjusting at first, but this is worth the effort now rather than later. You can slowly start putting your baby down sooner and sooner to develop this skill.

This stage can be tricky because your baby is still young and may fall asleep feeding quite often. This is why I mention starting to work on this now and it may not work each time and that's okay.

If you aren't already, begin using a sleeping phrase each time you put your child to sleep.

This can be a song or a phase such as:
"It's time to sleep little one, I love you. Good night."

Having a consistent sleeping phrase is a positive sleep prop to begin using to help your child know when it's time to sleep.

Milestones and regressions

The first few months of your baby's life brings a lot of changes, both mentally and physically. Baby's brain is undergoing a lot of development and their body is keeping up. There's also a sleep regression around the four month mark. Some babies can start showing signs of this around three and a half months old. This is a big change for your baby as his sleep cycles are becoming more like an adult's. You may notice your baby doesn't take long naps or is easily woken now. You may also notice that your child needs more help falling asleep.

MENTAL LEAP # 2: Leap 2 happens around 8 weeks and is all about pattern recognition. Your baby may start to take notice of small patterns, like lights and noises, which signal a big progression in mental development.

MENTAL LEAP # 3: Around 11 or 12 weeks, your baby will experience leap 3 — organization. While week 8 brought a lot of physical movement progression, around 12 weeks, your baby is able to perceive smooth transitions in sound, movement, light, taste, smell, and texture, but all still very simple.

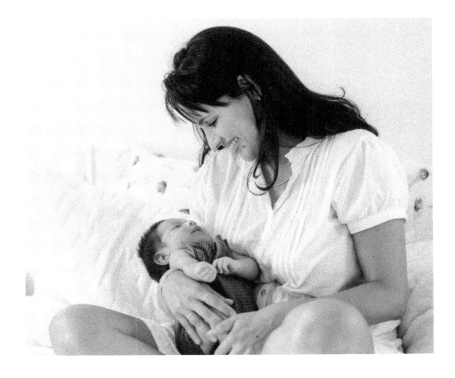

Between birth and three months, these are some of the changes baby experiences:

MOTOR SKILLS
- While lying on their tummy, your baby tries to push up on their arms
- While lying on their tummy, baby lifts and holds head up
- Can open and close fists
- Able to move hand to mouth
- Moves arms and legs off of surface when excited

SENSORY SKILLS
- While lying on back, tries to reach for a toy held above their chest
- While lying on back, visually tracks a toy moving from side to side
- While lying on back, keeps head centred to watch moving objects
- Able to calm down with rocking, touching, or gentle sounds

COMMUNICATION SKILLS
- Quiets or smiles in response to sounds or voices
- Turns head towards noises
- Shows interest in faces
- Makes eye contact
- Cries differently depending on needs (ex. hungry vs. tired)
- Coos and smiles

Self-regulation practice

Starting at around the end of three months old, you can slowly begin to encourage your baby when they become upset while trying something new. For example, during tummy time your child may fuss after a short time. Give them positive encouragement such as, "You are doing a great job of holding your head up! I know it's hard but keep trying!" Then wait five to ten seconds to see how she is doing. If she quiets down, let her be for a short time. If she continues to fuss, pick her up and tell her how great she did. Begin to extend this time as your child grows and start to notice what she does to distract herself.

3 – 6 months (12 – 24 weeks)

What to expect and what you can work on during this time

Your baby is changing at a rapid pace during this time. They will be growing and learning at a rapid pace and also going through several milestones. You will experience the four month sleep regression and that means more wakings, shorter naps, and some crankiness.

During this age, you will start to work away from sleep props and continue with a consistent bedtime routine.

Awake window

The awake window is anywhere between 1 ½ to 3 hours. Start using the Sleep Logs in the Appendix to find what works best for your baby.

Day and night schedule and routines

Keep in mind that this is a huge transition time for your little one. The best method when figuring out a schedule is to watch the clock and their sleepy cues, and have them sleep again within 1 ½ to 3 hours.

Remember, this is only an example of what your day might look like at this age with suggested nap times! The best method is to keep track of wake, eat, and sleep times to figure out the best schedule for you and your baby.

3-Month schedule example:

7:00 am	Wake and feed
7:30 am	Activity, such as tummy time or playing with you
8:30 am	Nap
10:00 am	Feed and play
11:30 am	Nap
1:00 pm	Feed and play
3:00 pm	Nap
4:00 pm	Feed and play
5:30 pm	Short nap
6:30 pm	Dinner
7:30 pm	Begin bedtime routine
8:00 – 8:30 pm	Goal to be asleep + night feeds

As your baby gets closer to six months old, they might be ready to drop a nap. Here's and example of what your day might look like closer to 6 months old:

6:30 am	Wake-up, feed, and play
7:45 am	Breakfast, some solids if starting
8:30 am	Nap (about 1 hour)
10:00 am	Feed and play
11:30 am	Nap (often 30 – 45 mins at this age)
1:00 pm	Feed
2:00 pm	Nap (often 30 – 45 mins at this age)
4:00 pm	Feed and play
4:30 pm	Short nap (30 mins)
5:00 pm	Dinner
6:00 pm	Bedtime routine
7:00 pm	Goal to be asleep + 1 to 2 night feeds

Night feeding tip:

If you have night feeds, have certain times that you feed so your child starts to have a pattern of when they wake for food. Many start to naturally sleep longer once they have a regular daytime schedule with good awake time windows and a good, consistent bedtime routine because they start to know what to do when it's sleepy time.

Sleep routines

Towards the end of six months, it's important to have a consistent bedtime routine in place. This routine should take no longer than 30 to 40 minutes. If the bath takes longer than that, consider that the bedtime routine starts after the bath.

- Bath (if giving that night)
- PJ's and diaper
- Feed (keeping baby awake)
- Brush teeth, if starting
- One to two calm books or calm songs
- Bed

Sleep props and sleeping phrase

Towards the end of six months, it's a good idea to work away from feeding to sleep and even stopping with the pacifier. These are the two harder sleep props to stop using and the sooner you begin to work on it, the better. It only gets harder to change these two as your baby gets older, more aware, and has more of a habit of using these to sleep.

If you haven't started with a sleeping phrase, this is a great time to begin. It is a source of comfort for them to hear the same repetitive phrase and be reminded of what they need to do. I recommend developing a sleeping phrase that is a short sentence or two, comforting, and relaxing. An example would be:

– *It's time to lay your head on your pillow and close your eyes because it's night-night time.*

– *Grab your teddy, lay your head down and relax your body; it's sleepy-time.*

Read more about developing your sleeping phrase on page 50.

Milestones and regressions

During this period, your baby is becoming more active and starting to use his hands more. You may even hear some strange noises coming from him as he starts to discover his voice. Around this time, your baby also goes through two more mental leaps. Remember, each baby will go through these milestones at different times and these are only general guidelines.

There's also a sleep regression around the four month mark. Some babies can start showing signs of this around three and a half months old. This is a big change for your baby as his sleep cycles are becoming more like an adult's. You may notice your baby doesn't take long naps or is easily woken now. You may also notice that your child needs more help falling asleep. Remember, although difficult, your baby is developing right on time if you're seeing this! Try to stay as consistent as possible but know you might have to help your baby fall asleep during this time. If the phase continues for longer than four weeks, look to see if your baby is relying on a sleep prop. You can review sleep props on page 46.

MENTAL LEAP # 4: In the last leap, we saw the perception of smooth transitions in sound, movement, light, taste, smell, and texture in a very simple manner. But around week 19 — sometimes between 18 and 20 — your baby begins to understand the world around him or her much better and can comprehend more complex situations.

Aside from these, baby has also learned some new skills:

MOTOR SKILLS
- Uses hands to support self while sitting
- Rolls from back to tummy and tummy to back
- While standing and supported, can hold entire weight on legs
- Reaches for things nearby when on tummy
- Reaches to play with feet while lying on back

SENSORY SKILLS
- Uses both hands to play with toys
- Happy when not tired or hungry
- Explores mouth — brings hands and objects to
- Is not upset or disturbed by everyday sounds

COMMUNICATION SKILLS
- Reacts to sudden noises or sounds
- Listens and responds when spoken to
- Babbles
- Uses babbling to get attention
- Makes different kinds of sounds to express feelings
- Notices toys that make sounds

Self-regulation practice

Slowly begin to encourage your baby when he becomes upset while trying something new. For example, during tummy time your child may fuss after a short time. Give him positive encouragement such as, "You are doing a great job of holding your head up! I know it's hard but keep trying!" Then wait five to ten seconds to see how he is doing. If he quiets down, let them be for a short time. If he continues to fuss, pick him up and tell him how great he did. Begin to extend this time as your child grows and starts to notice what he does to distract himself. The same applies to your child trying to crawl, walk, learn how to eat, or play with

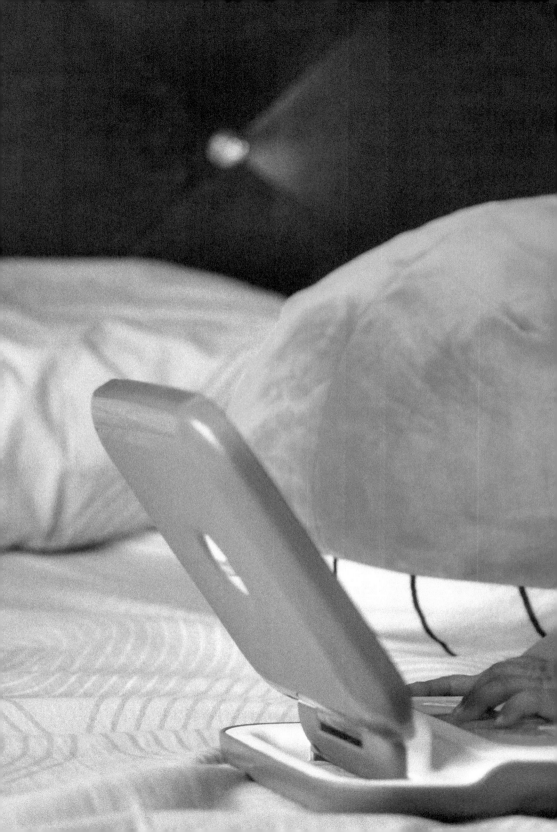

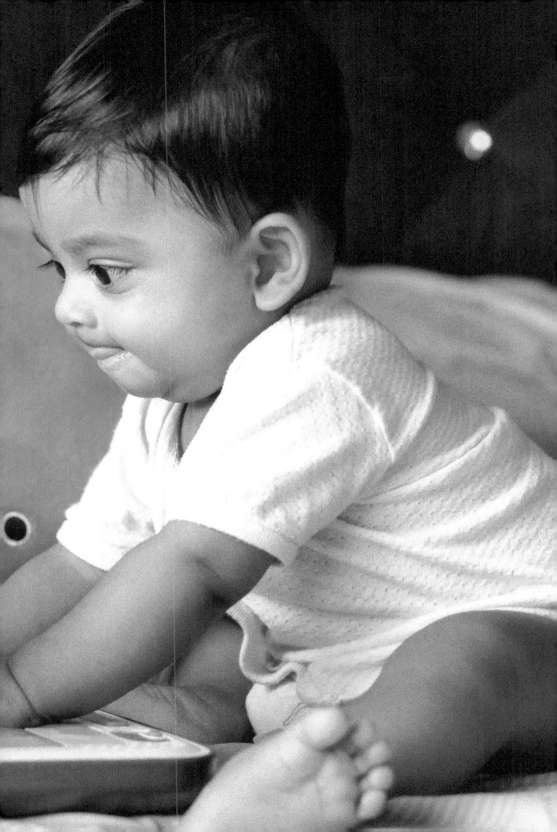

a new toy. Give them encouragement and time to work on the skill before you rush in to help.

Allow your child to have a little time in his crib once he wakes up from a nap. If you hear him, give him positive encouragement and tell him you'll be there soon. Wait (start with 10 seconds to 30 seconds) and then go in. This will let him know that it's ok to be in his crib. Begin to extend this time a little as your child grows. They don't need to be there for long, just enough to start finding a way to distract themself. When you come in, be sure to be excited, encouraging, and happy to see him. Tell them what a great job they did!

6 – 8 months (24 – 32 weeks)

What to expect and what you can work on during this time

Around six to seven months, babies are likely still on three naps, but soon will be dropping another nap. You may have days where your baby takes three naps and others two naps. On the two nap days, bedtime becomes earlier, especially on days where a third nap doesn't happen. Naps should be no later than 4 – 4:30 pm and bedtime should be no later than 2 – 3 hours after waking (7 – 7:30 pm).

Awake window

Awake time window is around 2 $\frac{1}{2}$ to 3 $\frac{1}{2}$ hours.

Day and night schedule and routines

Remember, this is only an example of what your day might look like at this age with suggested nap times! The best method is to keep track of wake, eat, and sleep times to figure out the best schedule for you. Once your baby wakes, be sure to watch the clock and their sleepy cues. Naps may vary from two to three naps per day depending on the length of the naps. Use the Nap logs in the Appendix to keep track of what works for your baby.

By now you probably have been feeding on a consistent schedule and some babies like little snacks all day long, while others like bigger meals. Feeding times will no longer be listed since this may vary from child to child.

THREE NAP SCHEDULE

7:00 am	Wake and breakfast (eat, play, snack)
9:00/9:30 am	Morning nap (using a nap routine)
12:00/12:30 pm	Midday nap (using a nap routine)
3:00 pm	Afternoon nap
6:15/6:30 pm	Begin bedtime routine
7:00 pm	Bed and goal to be asleep + one possible night feed

NIGHT FEEDING TIP:

If you have night feeds, have certain times that you feed so that your child starts to have a pattern of when they wake for food, if needed. Many start to naturally sleep longer once they have a regular daytime schedule with good awake time windows and a good, consistent bedtime routine because they start to know what to do when it's sleepy time.

TWO NAP SCHEDULE

7:00 am	Wake
9:30/10:00 am	Morning nap (using nap routine)
2:00 pm	Afternoon nap (using nap routine)
6:15/6:30 pm	Begin bedtime routine
7:00 pm	Bed with goal of being asleep + one possible night feed

Sleep routines

Around six months, it's important to have a consistent bedtime routine in place. This routine should take no longer than 30 to 40 minutes. If the bath takes longer than that, consider that the bedtime routine starts after the bath.

- Bath (if giving that night)
- PJ's and diaper
- Feed (while keeping baby awake)
- Brush teeth
- One to two calm books or calm songs
- Bed

Sleep props and sleeping phrase

If you haven't begun to work away from feeding to sleep and stopping with the pacifier, it's time to do that now if you are struggling with sleepless nights. These are the two harder sleep props to stop using and the sooner you begin to work on it, the better. It only gets harder to change these two as your baby gets older, more aware, and has more of a habit of using these to sleep.

If you are feeding your baby to sleep, you may notice he wakes up more often and has a harder time falling asleep if you stop feeding before he is in a deep sleep. Many will also get more energy even if they are just a little sleepy during this time. Be sure to feed in a bright room and keep them awake during this time.

If you haven't started with a sleeping phrase, this is a great time to begin. It is a source of comfort for them to hear the same repetitive phrase and be reminded of what they need to do. I recommend developing a sleeping phrase that is a short sentence or two, comforting, and relaxing. Examples would be:

– *It's time to lay your head on your pillow and close your eyes because it's night-night time."*
– *Grab your teddy, lay your head down and relax your body; it's sleepy-time."*

Milestones and regressions

This age is where your baby starts to need a constant eye. Crawling is one of the trademark milestones in this stage, so once they figure out how to move, you're going to have to make sure you keep up. If you haven't baby-proofed your home yet, this is the time you'll want to get on that!

Around the six month mark you may notice that your child has a phase of difficult sleep. While there isn't a full sleep regression at this age, it could be due to a growth spurt around this time. Closer to the eight to ten month mark is when you will notice your child going through a sleep regression and this is due to the leaps in development she is making. Clear signs will be increased crankiness, clinginess, and crying.

MENTAL LEAP # 5: Leap 5 generally happens around 26 weeks and involves an increased understanding of the relationships around her. As she starts to become more mobile, she can now understand distance between objects. Their world has transformed from a little place to one that's quite large.

MENTAL LEAP # 6: Around 37 weeks, sometimes 36 – 40, baby's curiosity peaks as he or she attempts to do new things. They're now at a stage where they can recognize certain objects, animals, sensations, and people who belong in the same group or category; they are learning about differences and similarities. For example, bananas taste, look, and feel different than spinach.

In addition to these distinctions, baby also learns some new skills:

MOTOR SKILLS
- Able to sit without support
- Sits and reaches for objects or toys without falling
- Can move from tummy or back to sit
- Alternate leg and arm movements (crawling)
- Picks up head and pushes through elbows during tummy time
- Turns head to visually track objects
- Shows more control while rolling and sitting
- Picks up small objects with hands

SENSORY SKILLS
- Enjoys a variety of movements (bouncing, rocking, etc.)
- Explores objects with both hands and mouth
- Experiments with force needed to pick different objects up
- Focuses on close and distant objects
- Observes environment from several positions (lying on back, sitting, crawling, assisted standing)

COMMUNICATION SKILLS
- Increased variety of sounds while babbling
- Looks at people and objects when named
- Recognizes sound of own name
- Participates in two-way communication
- Shows recognition of commonly used words
- Uses simple gestures (ex. shakes head for no)
- Imitates sounds

Self-regulation practice

You may notice that your child starts to get more vocal if he or she can't do something or get something right away. You can work on self-regulation by giving your child positive encouragement such as, "You are doing a great job! I know it's hard but keep trying!" Wait 30 seconds to one minute to see how they are doing. If they quiet down, let them be for a short time. If they continue to fuss, pick them up and tell them how great they did. Keep extending this time as your child grows and start to notice what they do to distract himself.

The same applies to your child trying to crawl, walk, learn to eat, or play with a new toy. Give them encouragement and time to work on the skill before you rush in to help.

Allow your child to have a little time in their crib once she wakes up from a nap. If you hear her wake up, give her positive encouragement and tell her you'll be there soon. Wait, starting with 30 seconds to one minute, and then go in. This will let her begin to know that it's okay to be in her crib. Begin to extend this time a little as your child grows. They don't need to be there for long, just enough to start finding a way to distract themself. When you come in, be sure to be excited, encouraging, and happy to see them. Tell her what a great job she did!

8 – 12 months (32 – 48 weeks)

What to expect and what you can work on during this time

At this age, your baby will be transiting from three to two naps. It might feel like a continuous sleep regression during this stage and even if your child refuses a nap, don't rush to drop that nap right away! The last nap should end around 4:30 pm with bedtime being about 3 hours after waking. Bedtime should be no later than 7 – 8 pm. If your baby starts to wake more frequently at night, scale the bedtime back a little earlier or look at any sleeping props that you might be using to help your child fall asleep.

Awake window

Awake time window can be anywhere between 2 ½ to 4 hours.

Day and night schedule and routines

Remember, this is only an example of what your day might look like at this age with suggested nap times for two or three naps. It's important to watch your baby's sleeping cues, along with their awake window, but the timing of the naps will become more important at this age because they need a consistent sleep and awake pattern in their body to be ready for sleeping at night.

THREE NAP SCHEDULE

7:00 am	Wake and breakfast (eat, play, (snack), sleep routine)
9:00/9:30 am	Morning nap (using a nap routine)
12:00/12:30 pm	Midday nap (using a nap routine)
3:00 pm	Afternoon nap
6:15/6:30 pm	Begin bedtime routine
7:00 pm	Bed and goal to be asleep + one possible night feed

Night feeding tip:

If you have night feeds, decide on one certain time that you feed so that your child starts to have a pattern of when to wake for food, if your child needs a night feeding. Many start to naturally sleep longer once they have a regular daytime schedule with good awake time windows and a good, consistent bedtime routine because they start to know what to do when it's sleepy time.

You might wonder if more solids will help your baby sleep. Most will say that having a full tummy will prevent wakings, and while it's important that your child is full before bed, if they wake up often throughout the night, there's generally an underlying reason as to why and more food won't fix that. Look to see if your child is using feeding to sleep as a way to fall back to sleep. Then you'll know why he is waking, as he is using it as a way to help fall asleep.

TWO NAP SCHEDULE

7:00 am	Wake
9:30/10:00 am	Morning nap (using nap routine)
2:00 pm	Afternoon nap (using nap routine)
6:15/6:30 pm	Begin bedtime routine
7:00 pm	Bed with goal of being asleep + one possible night feed

Sleep routines

At this age it's important to have a consistent bedtime routine in place. This routine should take no longer than 30 to 40 minutes. If the bath takes longer than that, consider that the bedtime routine starts after the bath. The final feeding before bedtime is now sooner than in previous routines. It's good to start moving the final feeding to a little earlier in the routine to help disassociate feeding and sleep.

- Bath (if giving that night)
- Feed (no drowsiness during the feed)
- PJ's and diaper
- Brush teeth
- One to two calm books or calm songs
- Bed

Sleep props and sleeping phrase

If you haven't begun to work away from feeding to sleep and stopping with the pacifier, it's time to do that now if you are struggling with sleepless nights. These are the two harder sleep props to stop using and the sooner you begin to work on it, the better. It only gets harder to change these two as your baby gets older, more aware, and has more of a habit of using these to sleep.

If you are feeding your baby to sleep, you may notice they wake up more and have a harder time falling asleep if you stop feeding and they aren't in a deep sleep. Many will also get more energy even if they are just a little sleepy during this time. Be sure to feed in a bright room and keep them awake during this time.

If you haven't started with a sleeping phrase, this is a great time to begin. It is a source of comfort for them to hear the same repetitive phrase and be reminded of what they need to do. I recommend developing a sleeping phrase that is a short sentence or two, comforting, and relaxing. Examples would be:

– *It's time to lay your head on your pillow and close your eyes because it's night-night time.*
– *Grab your teddy, lay your head down and relax your body; it's sleepy-time.*

Milestones and regressions

At this point in time, your baby is starting to look and act more like a toddler, but in many ways, she is still a baby. While these are some of the big milestones your baby is going to hit, every baby will experience them at a different time. There is no set time to which these events should occur, so whether your baby hits one during the proper stage or not, the important thing to remember is that your baby is always moving forward in her development.

This timeframe might feel like a continuous sleep regression since there is a lot going on in your child's brain and body, resulting in sleep disruptions. You might see your child have some sleep troubles sometime between 8 – 10 months and again around their first birthday. Try to stay as consistent as you can but don't be surprised if you need to help your child for a short period of time to fall asleep. You'll recognize the regression and leap period with increased crying, crankiness, and wanting to be close to you. These time periods may last anywhere from two to six weeks. If you have a long period of time with sleep troubles, take a look at how much you are helping your child fall asleep.

MENTAL LEAP # 7: Around 46 weeks, baby's mess making abilities seem to take a little bit of a turn as she starts to put things together now. This is a time when they start to discover sequencing — she must do things in a certain order to accomplish something.

There's also another new set of motor, sensory, and communication skills:

MOTOR SKILLS

- Pulls self to stand and uses furniture to move
- Can stand and take several steps alone
- Moves in and out of various positions
- Maintains balance
- Claps hands
- Can release objects into container with large opening
- Can pick up small objects
- Begins to feed themselves

SENSORY SKILLS

- Enjoys listening to music
- Explores toys with hands, fingers, and mouth
- Crawls to distant people or objects

COMMUNICATION SKILLS

- Can use 'mama' or 'dada' in proper context
- Responds to simple directions (ex. come here)
- Produces long strings of babble
- Says first words
- Imitates speech sounds
- Babble has rhythms and sounds of speech
- Pays attention to where you are looking or pointing
- Responds to "no"
- Begins to use hand movements to communicate wants and needs (ex. reaches to be picked up)

At this point, your baby has gone through a tremendous amount of change, both physically and mentally. After baby's first year, there are still three mental leaps he will make:

MENTAL LEAP # 8: Just after your baby's first birthday, around 55 weeks, he or she will go through yet another leap — this one is exploring the world of programs. While the previous leap was about putting things in the correct order, this one takes an if-then approach; the next event or sequence that happens depends on what just happened.

Self-regulation practice

You may notice that your child starts to get more vocal if he can't do something or get something right away. You can work on self-regulation by giving him positive encouragement such as, "You are doing a great job of trying to get that toy! I know it's hard but keep trying!" Wait one minute to see how he is doing. If he quiets down, let him be for a short time. If he continues to fuss, pick him up and tell him how great he did. Keep extending this time as your child grows and starts to notice what he does to distract himself.

The same applies to your child trying to crawl, walk, learn how to eat, or play with a new toy. Give her encouragement and time to work on the skill before you rush in to help.

Allow your child to have a little time in her crib once she wakes up from a nap. If you hear her, give her positive encouragement and tell her you'll be there soon. Wait, starting with one minute, and then go in. This will let her begin to know that it's ok to be in her crib. Begin to extend this time a little as your child grows. They don't need to be there for long, just enough to start finding a way to distract themself. When you come in, be sure to be excited, encouraging, and happy to see them. Tell her what a great job she did!

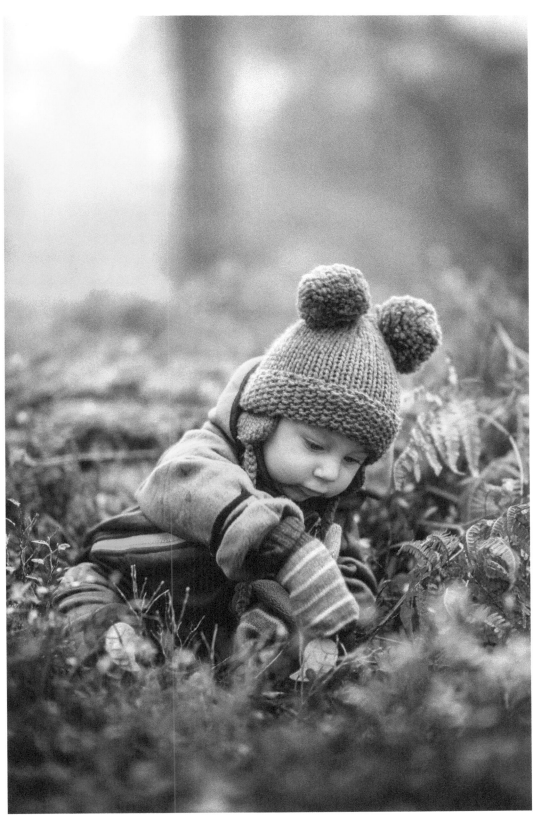

13 – 18 months

What to expect and what you can work on during this time

At this age, your baby is likely taking two naps. There's a sleep regression during this stage and even if your child refuses a nap, don't rush to drop the second nap! The longer you can hold off on the transition to a single nap, the smoother it will be. As with before, the last nap should end around 4pm with bedtime being 3 – 4 hours after waking. Bedtime should be no later than 7 – 8 pm. If your baby starts to wake more frequently at night, scale the bedtime back a little earlier or look at any sleeping props that you might be using to help your child fall asleep.

For babies that have successfully transitioned to a single nap, the morning nap should be pushed later until it happens around noon. At this point, you want to put your baby to sleep about 4 1/2 – 5 hours after waking.

Awake window

Awake window is around 4 1/2 – 5 hours.

Day and night schedule and routines

Remember, this is only an example of what your day might look like at this age with a suggested nap time. Some children may drop their second nap around 15 to 18 months, but keep in mind that there is a sleep regression during this period. Try to keep the second nap as long as possible, even if some days your child takes one nap and then on other days takes two naps.

TWO NAP SCHEDULE

7:00 am	Wake
9:30/10:00 am	Morning nap (using nap routine)
2:00 pm	Afternoon nap (using nap routine)
6:15/6:30 pm	Begin bedtime routine
7:00 pm	Bed with goal of being asleep

ONE NAP SCHEDULE

7:00 am	Wake
11:30/12:00 pm	Afternoon nap (using nap routine)
6:15/6:30 pm	Begin bedtime routine
7:00 pm	Bed with goal of being asleep

Sleep routines

Whatever your bedtime routine is, your toddler will probably insist that it be the same every night, which is great! Just don't allow rituals to become too long or complicated, ideally they should be around 30 to 40 minutes. Whenever possible, let your toddler make bedtime choices within the routine: which pajamas to wear, which stuffed animal to take to bed, or what music to play. This gives your little one a sense of control. A typical routine at this age may look like:

(If the bath takes longer, consider that the bedtime routine starts after the bath.)
- Feeding or a snack
- Bath (if giving that night)
- PJ's and diaper
- Brush teeth
- One to two calm books or calm songs
- Bed

Sleep props and sleeping phrase

If you haven't begun to work away from feeding to sleep and stopping with the pacifier, it's time to do that now if you are struggling with sleepless nights. These are the two harder sleep props to stop using and the sooner you begin to work on it, the better. It only gets harder to change these two as your baby gets older, more aware, and has more of a habit of using these to sleep.

If you are feeding your baby to sleep, you may notice they wake up more and have a harder time falling asleep if you stop feeding and they aren't in a deep sleep. Many will also get more energy even if they are just a little sleepy during this time. Be sure to feed in a bright room and keep them awake during this time.

If you haven't started with a sleeping phrase, it's time to begin. It is a source of comfort for them to hear the same repetitive phrase and be reminded of what they need to do. I recommend developing a sleeping phrase that is a short sentence or two, comforting, and relaxing. Examples would be:

– *It's time to lay your head on your pillow and close your eyes because it's night-night time."*
– *Grab your teddy, lay your head down and relax your body; it's sleepy-time."*

Milestones and regressions

There are so many wonderful things happening at this age but it also comes with another sleep regression around 15 – 18 months old. You'll recognize the regression and leap period with increased crying, crankiness, and wanting to be close to you. Try to stay as consistent as you can but don't be surprised if you need to help your child for a short period of time to fall asleep. These time periods may last anywhere from two to six weeks. If you have a long period of time with sleep troubles, take a look at how much you are helping your child fall asleep.

MENTAL LEAP # 9: Mental leap 9 happens around 64 weeks and is all about your baby's ability to change the programs they have learned thus far. Here's some of what baby is learning:

- Increased skillfulness with things and language
- Imitates others
- Practices emotions
- Starts to think ahead
- Starts to be 'aggressive'
- Starts experimenting with 'yes' and 'no'
- Learns how to get someone to do something for him or her
- Learns to do something together

MENTAL LEAP # 10: While there are only 10 leaps studied and listed, your child will continue to have developmental leaps throughout their child-hood. The brain doesn't reach maturity until around age 25! Thus said, leap 10 happens around 75 weeks (17 months) where your toddler learns a new ability to perceive and handle "systems." He or she now under-stands the world of principles and can choose how he or she wants to be: honest, helpful, patient, careful, etc.

While there is more development that your baby will go through, these are the milestones that have been researched. Continue watching and enjoying your child's growth and development!

Self-regulation practice

You may notice that your child starts to get more vocal if they can't do something or get something right away. You can work on self-regulation by giving them positive encouragement such as, "You are doing a great job! I know it's hard but keep trying!" Wait a minute or two to see how they are doing. If they quiet down, let them be for a short time. If they continue to fuss, pick them up and tell them how great they did. Keep extending this time as your child grows and start to notice what they do to distract themself.

The same applies to your child trying to crawl, walk, learn how to eat, or play with a new toy. Give them encouragement and time to work on the skill before you rush in to help.

Allow your child to have a little time in their crib once they wake up from a nap. If you hear them, give them positive encouragement and tell them you'll be there soon. Wait, starting with one minute, and then go in. This will let them begin to know that it's ok to be in their crib. Begin to extend this time a little as your child grows. They don't need to be there for long, just enough to start finding a way to distract themself. When you come in, be sure to be excited, encouraging, and happy to see them. Tell them what a great job they did!

It's also a good idea to start with what I call loving boundaries. Rules are often thought as too hard for young kids, but it's a good idea to have some loving boundaries as to what you do in your home. At this age there are a lot of feelings and emotions that kids can't explain yet. Sometimes it comes out as anger, hitting, yelling, and frustration and it's hard for them to understand why they feel this way. It can be a frustrating time for you and your child, but try to remember that all children mean well and they need guidance from us adults.

One common question I often get asked is why a child has a melt-down over a simple question you ask them or that they often seem frustrated or angry. My first question back to them is, of course, about sleep, but then I talk about loving boundaries. It comes down to the child feeling overwhelmed with the amount of options they have. We might think that allowing our children to make their own decisions is a great thing, and it is, to an extent, but the problem is that children can often feel overwhelmed by the amount of choices they have to choose from. This is where loving boundaries come into play. Instead of deciding everything for them and not giving them a choice at all verses offering them too many choices, you offer only a couple of options.

Loving boundaries mean you offer two options instead of offering up every choice. You can ask, "Would you like the blue or the green one?" instead of "Which cup do you want?" and there are too many colors for your child to choose from, so they end up feeling frustrated because they can't decide. Another example is when you choose a book at bedtime. You choose two books and then ask them which book they want to read tonight. It limits arguments, pushing to read five different books, or a frustrated child who can't decide which book to read.

For more information on this topic, I highly recommend reading *How To Talk So Little Kids Will Listen : A Survival Guide to Life with Children Ages 2 – 7* by Joanna Faber and Julie King. It's a great resource for communication skills with kids during the tricky years!

2 – 5 years

What to expect and what you can work on during this time

19 MONTHS – 3 YEARS: By this age, your little one should be on a consistent one nap a day schedule, happening around the middle of the day. Any nap should end by 4pm at the latest and your child should be put to bed no later than 4 ½ – 5 hours after waking, usually around 7 – 8 pm.

Every child is different when it comes to napping and some drop their nap around 2 years old. You'll know your child is ready to stop with their nap when they struggle to fall asleep at bedtime or start having a hard time sleeping at night when it hasn't been a problem.

3 YEARS + : Many children drop their last nap around 3 years. While a nap is not happening, it's important to give your child a period of quiet time where they are resting to allow them to regroup and recharge. Since your child is not having a nap, a consistent bedtime is a must. At 3 – 5 years, they still need 11 – 13 hours of sleep a night, so bedtime should be around 6 – 8 pm timeframe. If at 8 pm it's difficult to get your child to sleep, try bedtime a bit earlier because you've likely missed the optimal window and he is now overtired.

Awake window

Awake time increases to 4 to 6 hours by 2 years-old.

Day and night schedule and routines

NOOO! Are you hearing this often nowadays? What a time for learning independence, but one thing is for sure, sleeping is not to be forgotten. It may seem like your child has a lot of energy, but getting enough sleep is crucial at this age. If you are dealing with a cranky toddler, think about how much sleep she is getting. If your child is ready to drop a nap, check the dropping a nap section on page 62 for more info.

TWO NAP SCHEDULE

7:00 am	Wake
9:30/10:00 am	Morning nap (using nap routine)
2:00 pm	Afternoon nap (using nap routine)
6:15/6:30 pm	Begin bedtime routine
7:00 pm	Bed with goal of being asleep

Dropping another nap varies from child to child. If your child is not sleeping for the afternoon nap or struggling to sleep through the night and that hasn't been an issue, then it's time to consider going to a one nap schedule.

ONE NAP SCHEDULE

7:00 am	Wake
12:00 pm	Afternoon nap (using nap routine)
6:15/6:30 pm	Begin bedtime routine
7:00 pm	Bed with goal of being asleep

Sleep routines

Whatever your bedtime routine is, your toddler will probably insist that it be the same every night. Just don't allow rituals to become too long or complicated, ideally they should be around 30 to 40 minutes. Whenever possible, let your toddler make bedtime choices within the routine:

which pajamas to wear, which stuffed animal to take to bed, or what music to play. This gives your little one a sense of control.

A typical routine at this age may look like:
(If the bath takes longer than 30 minutes, consider that the bedtime routine starts after the bath.)
- Feeding or a snack
- Bath (if giving that night)
- PJ's and diaper
- Brush teeth
- One to two calm books or calm songs
- Bed

Sleep props and sleeping phrase

If you haven't begun to work away from feeding to sleep and stopping with the pacifier, it's time to do that now if you are struggling with sleepless nights. These are the two harder sleep props to stop using and the sooner you begin to work on it, the better. It only gets harder to change these two as your baby gets older, more aware, and has more of a habit of using these to sleep.

If you are feeding your child to sleep, you may notice they wake up more and have a harder time falling asleep if you stop feeding and they aren't in a deep sleep. Many will also get more energy even if they are just a little sleepy during this time. Be sure to feed in a bright room and keep them awake during this time.

If you haven't started with a sleeping phrase, it's time to begin. It is a source of comfort for them to hear the same repetitive phrase and be reminded of what they need to do. I recommend developing a sleeping phrase that is a short sentence or two, comforting, and relaxing. Examples would be:

– *It's time to lay your head on your pillow and close your eyes because it's night-night time.*
– *Grab your teddy, lay your head down and relax your body; it's sleepy-time.*

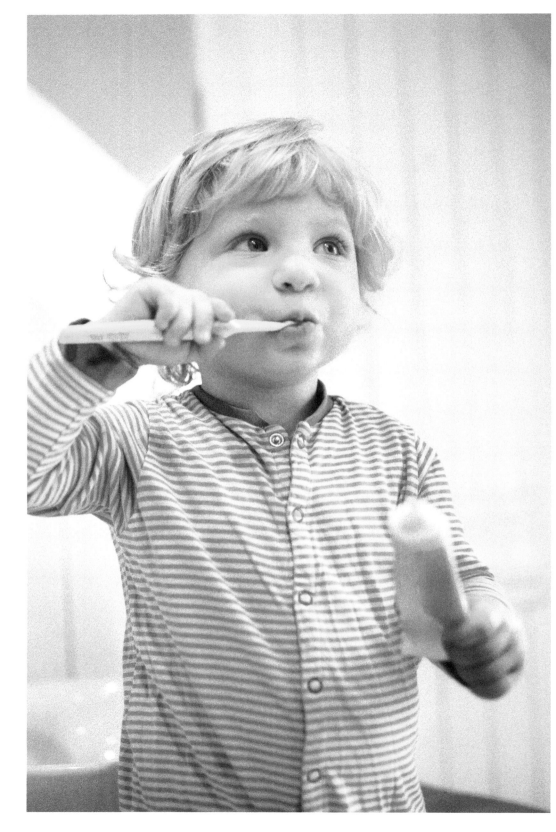

Milestones and regressions

Expect another regression time around your child's second birthday. Stay as consistent as possible with those strong two-year old demands! While there are only 10 leaps studied and listed, your child will continue to have developmental leaps throughout their childhood. The brain doesn't reach maturity until around age 25!

- There's so much going on in toddler development at this stage.
- Expect big feelings, tantrums, simple sentences, pretend play, independence, new thinking skills and much more.
- Talking and listening, reading, working on everyday skills, and cooking together are good for development.

Self-regulation practice

You can work on self-regulation by giving them positive encouragement if they are struggling with something such as, "You are doing a great job of playing with that toy! I know it's hard to figure it out but keep trying!" Wait one to two minutes to see how they are doing. If they quiet down, let them be for a short time. If they continue to fuss, go over to them and tell them how great they did. Keep extending this time as your child grows and start to notice what they do to distract themself. Give them encouragement and time to work on the skill before you rush in to help.

Allow your child to have a little time in their crib once they wake up from a nap. If you hear them, give them positive encouragement and tell them you'll be there soon. Wait, starting with one to two minutes, and then go in. This will let them begin to know that it's ok to be in their crib. Begin to extend this time a little as your child grows. They don't need to be there for long, just enough to start finding a way to distract themself. When you come in, be sure to be excited, encouraging, and happy to see them. Tell them what a great job they did!

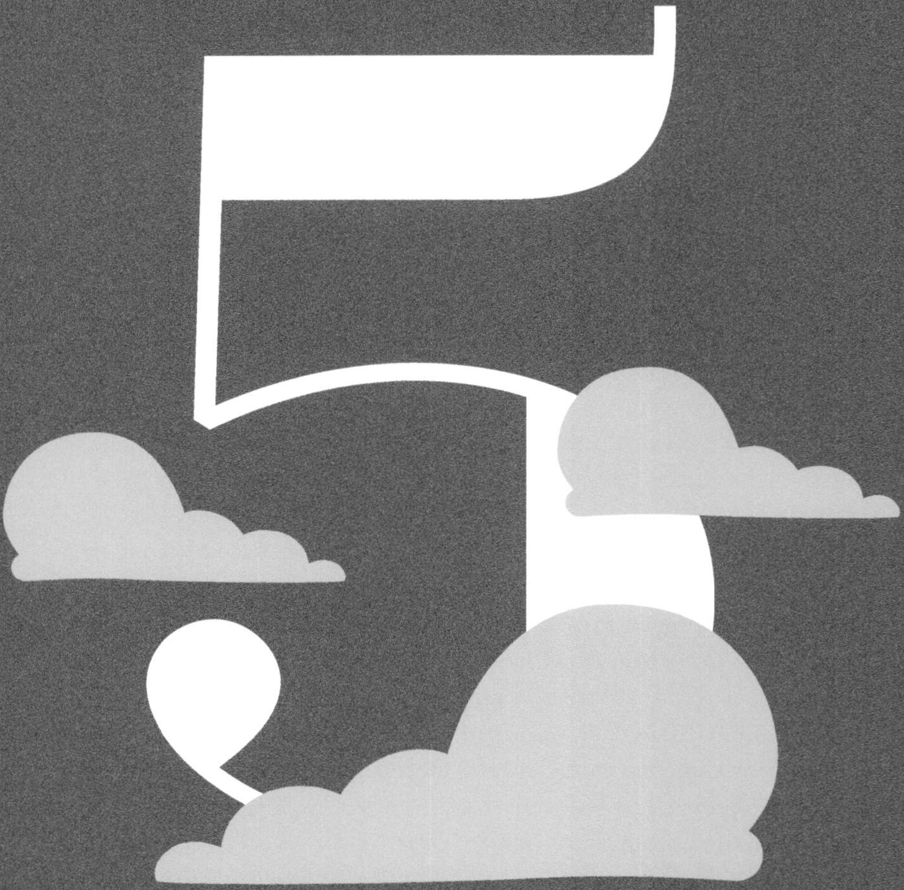
5

Steps towards more sleep

What is sleep training?

There isn't one way to sleep train and in fact, any type of changes or skills you are helping your child learn are considered "sleep training". The concept of training your baby to sleep may even sound a little strange to you. Surely, a child should enjoy and benefit from natural sleep rather than be "trained," right? That's what I thought in the beginning, too! Then I had a baby who needed help understanding when it was time to sleep and what that feeling meant in her body. The thing about training your child is that it can actually help them, and you, to get the right amount of restful sleep. It's a way of protecting your baby and keeping them healthy and happy. Training or practicing healthy sleep habits is no different than your baby learning how to eat, go potty, or crawl on their own. Each takes time, practice, and patience. Sleep training should be called sleep learning instead!

Sleep training is simply a way for you to help your child understand how to sleep, so he gets the rest he needs. If your child still seems reluctant to sleep for longer periods, do not worry. Every child and family is different as to what approach fits them best.

What works in one home may not work in another. There are different methods to help your baby sleep, so let's go over some of the most common terms when it comes to sleep training.

The three main baby sleep training methods

You will see several sleep training methods mentioned by experts. No one method is best, you simply need to find the method that works in your situation. Let's take a look at the three main methods so that you can understand the terms better.

1 **NO TEARS** This method tries to reduce crying to a minimum. Now, I should mention that there probably won't be "no tears" but the goal is to have as few as possible. You will be helping your child quite a bit to fall asleep and as soon as your baby cries, you should comfort and soothe them immediately. The problem you may find is that some babies tend to be more attention seeking than others. If your baby knows you will come if they cry, training them to sleep could be a long process. You will need a lot of patience and time using this method. For older children, I find this method to be very difficult because it takes a long time to see results. Maybe your baby isn't crying, but you are because you are so tired and don't have any patience left. It can take anywhere from a couple of weeks to a month before you might see changes. This method works best for babies six months and under.

2 **FADING METHOD** This method of baby sleep training is popular with a lot of parents and one that has a nice balance of learning and love. It involves moving further away from your child's crib each night as they fall asleep. They get used to you being at arm's length and then not being in the room, and it's a gradual process. Fading also involves checking in on your baby, but making it less obvious over time and eventually he or she is not even aware of your presence. You can expect to see improvements anywhere from three nights to a month with this method. This method is best starting from five months and up.

3 **CRY IT OUT** This method is as it sounds, but I should mention that this method has been changed over the years with advice to check on your child more often. This method is only advised for babies four months and older, although I don't think it's appropriate until six months old. To do this method, you place your baby in their crib and you leave the

room and return at regular intervals to help soothe. This does not mean that you should just leave your baby crying for hours, although some sleep programs do suggest this. If attempting this method, it's best to place your baby in his crib before he gets too tired. Let them be on their own for a while when you leave and go back to soothe them if necessary. In this method you do not pick your baby up; simply soothe him with your voice. This method can be difficult for some parents to manage. Although this is the method many pediatricians advise parents to use, I believe there are better ways to help a baby develop healthy sleep habits. This method may not suit all families. This method tends to have fairly quick results (you'll see changes within three days but you won't be finished) if you stick to it. Again, this method is advised for babies four months and older.

You may need to try different methods or a mix of the methods to find the one that works best for you and your baby. Do not simply expect that what worked for a previous child or a friend's child will work with the baby you are currently training to sleep. Be prepared to adapt and change routines and methods until you settle on what works the best. My best tip is to understand your child's temperament, decide on a method, make a plan, try it for one week, take notes, and use the sleep logs in the appendix to see any positive changes (even small ones), and then decide if it's working for you and your baby.

I also don't use the terms cry it out or no tears within the following plans. Remember, just because you choose a "no cry" method doesn't necessarily mean no tears, it means minimizing tears as much as possible! *There isn't any method that can promise "no tears" and if there was, wouldn't everyone use it!?* I find that term to be extremely misleading and then parents feel as if they have failed when it doesn't work. Some children are overstimulated with too much help and they will still be crying. The same goes for crying it out. Some children will be upset at first, but then do really well without parental help. Instead, I use these terms for the different methods:

- **HOLD & HELP**

  Works best for babies under six months. Works well for sensitive babies and babies with a strong sleep association.

- **FADING**

  Best for around five months and up and for any temperament type.

- **LEAVE & CHECK**

  Best for babies six months and older. Works well for strong willed babies or babies overstimulated by a parent's help.

Within the following sections, you will have different options to try. I would suggest starting with one method for a week before making a change. It can take a few days for your child to adjust to the new way, so don't expect things to magically change in one night.

Weeks 2 and 3

Before you begin weeks 2 and 3, be sure to have the check list in week 1 complete (page 73). The methods below are adapted to be parent-assisted methods and you have the ability to help your child learn new habits of falling asleep. You are your child's sleep guide from here on out and know that your actions will help you get towards your sleep goals as a family. Before you begin, choose an option or at least have a plan on how you'll adapt your approach to sleep training. *The best approach is to be as consistent as possible to help your child learn this new skill of sleep. It's also important to believe that this process will work! If you don't believe that this will work, you are more likely to not follow through on your plan.*

It's also important to note that I'd like you to reduce the number of activities you do during this time! You might need to skip a parent group, baby swim, or other activities if it interferes with learning this new skill. It's just short-term, you'll be back to normal soon! It's fine to continue the activities if they fit into your schedule without disrupting your new sleep schedule.

What to expect

There is no "one right way" to help a child learn how to sleep. Some children are more stimulated by the parent in the room, while other children are more calmed with the parent in the room during sleep training. Some parents are more reassured the more involved they are in the training; other parents find it easier to be as removed from the training as possible. As you are making changes to your child's sleep, you can expect a little push back because this is new to them. They will not fully understand why things are changing! Be calm, reassuring, and patient when making these changes because they most likely will not happen overnight.

The best way to use each method is to follow the outlined plan as close as possible. However, as a parent, you know what's best for your child, so modify as needed. Remember, changes aren't easy for a baby to go through, so expect there to be some tears — although not fun, it's totally normal when having to learn a new skill.

You're also probably wondering how much your child will cry and the answer is, it depends. It depends on your child's age, what their sleep prop is or has been, their temperament, are they in a leap or regression phase, and if their naps and awake windows are set up for their age. Working on all the elements in Week 1 will help reduce fuss at bedtime, but expect some upset since your baby is now being asked to do a completely new skill that they haven't done before – falling asleep more on their own. For example, if your child has been fed to sleep for eight months and now they are being asked to fall asleep on their own, of course they are upset, as they didn't know they wouldn't be fed to sleep forever! Of course it's confusing for them, having to do it on their own now. This will take some time to adjust, but believe that your child can do it!

There is no guarantee when your child will begin sleeping through the night or stop getting up a billion times before falling to sleep, but many children start improving the length of time they sleep within five days. *The fastest changes happen when you are consistent with the new routines.*

> The first days on the new schedule will be an adjustment for everyone. Please be patient and continue as consistency pays off.

Each of these methods builds a growth-promoting environment to help your child practice the skills to fall asleep by first helping her before she will do it alone. Change can be hard no matter what age you are, but giving guidance and support helps build trust. Keep in mind that even when making changes built around trust and guidance, there will still be an adaptation period that may come out as crankiness, sleeping worse, or sadness. Change can be challenging, but we never want it to be overwhelming for a child. If you are concerned about stress, review the section on page 81.

Expect crying will happen and it's not bad when making big changes, especially if you are there supporting your child.

Lastly, choose a start date. It's important to decide on a night to start your plan as "we'll try tonight" usually doesn't end up with much follow through, not to mention you'll experience more frustration than needed for both you and your child.

· · · · · SLEEP TASK · · · · ·

Use this chapter to start writing your plan and what's best for your family here. Be sure to choose a date that you will begin your new way of putting your child to sleep.

Your sleep goals

As with any changes in life, having a reason or a goal is important to help keep you on track. When you are adjusting to the first days of the plan, remember your sleep goals to help motivate you. You are doing this program for your child's health, your health, and to make family life less hectic! I would suggest writing these down and putting them in a place where you will see them regularly.

Some sample goals might be:
- Establish a sleep routine to help understand when it's time to sleep
- Work towards one to zero night wakings

· · · · · **SLEEP TASK** · · · · ·

We are working towards:

★

★

★

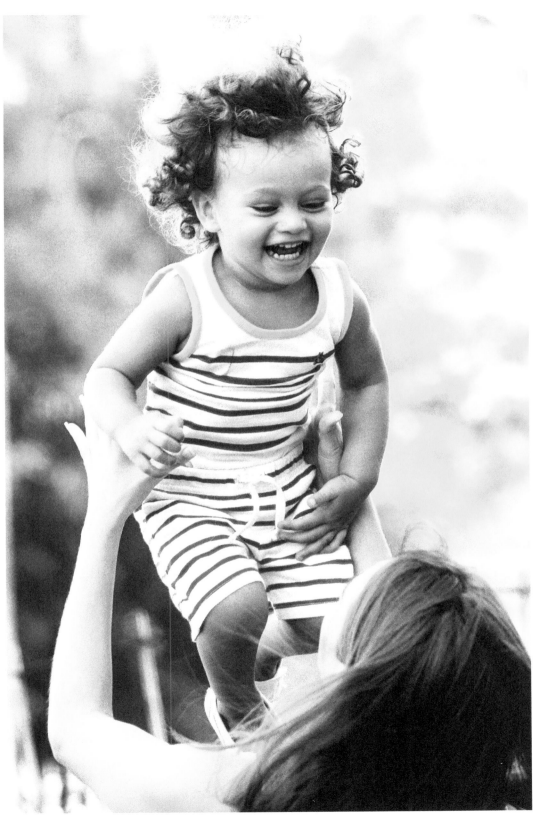

Sleeping is a skill

Sleeping truly is a skill. It's a skill that is important in many other areas of your baby's life, too, but it's a process to learn just like all skills. We give our babies time to learn how to crawl, eat with a spoon, interact with other children, so why don't we give them more time to learn how to sleep? Teaching is part of parenthood.

Some babies do sleep less, yes, it's true. And knowing your baby's sleep needs will help your baby be a much happier baby! You'll be surprised how a "fussy" baby begins to be easier once she starts sleeping more.

Happy sleep methods

Before you begin:

- Make sure you have completed Week 1 to help sleep happen more naturally.

- To prepare for the first several nights, read *Night 1 through 4*, *Night waking*, and *Crying* below before you begin.

- Use the resources in the Appendix to develop your sleep plan for your family. Be sure to use the Sleep Logs to track how your progress is going!

- You'll also find a sleep plan cheat sheet for the method you choose to use within the Appendix. This is a shortened version of the following methods to help remind you of what to do.

> **SLEEP TIP!** Decide which parent will start the plan. If the baby has been nursed to sleep, it's best if the other parent takes the first few nights. Both parents can be involved and you can switch who does what, but for the first few nights choose the parent that can calm your child easiest. Sometimes it's not the parent you think it will be!

Day 1

You'll do just as you have been the last few days by following your baby's awake time window or nap schedule, consistent routines, and making sure their room is ready for sleep. You'll put your baby to sleep as you have been doing for naps. You'll begin your sleep changes at bedtime.

Nights 1 through 4

Generally, the first night of changes will take about 45 minutes to one hour before your child falls asleep. Now, this is a general timeframe that I notice for most of my parents. It could go faster for you! If your child isn't sleeping after 45 minutes, take a minute to think about what you are doing. Are you helping your child too much and causing them frustration or overstimulation? Most of the time it takes longer because the child is not being allowed to work on the skill on their own. Believe your child can make these changes and give it a chance!

You'll begin Night 1 after you've done your bedtime routine, follow the steps below for the method you choose.

☆ HOLD & HELP
- After a cuddle and your baby is beginning to get sleepy, put your baby into his crib, give him some time to settle on his own.
- You can help your baby to sleep with touch, gentle rocking while they are laying down, singing or using your sleeping phrase.
- If your baby becomes upset, pick them up and help soothe for about two minutes. Then lay him back down.
- Repeat this process until your baby falls asleep.

☆ FADING
- Sit sideways in a chair next to your child's bed. You will sit sideways to the bed because we want to limit interaction and show that it's not play time but sleeping time.
- If your child is moving around or starts to fuss, say your sleeping phrase to help calm her. If your child doesn't need to hear the sleeping

phrase or if it makes her upset, just stay quiet. Be sure to stay calm yourself. It is important that you stay calm during this time, as we are making changes to your child's regular routine and you are her emotional guide.

- If your child can stand, you can lay them down. Give a few minutes in between if they stand up immediately. Lay them down *five times*, but after the fifth time, let them stand. You can try to coax them down by patting the mattress and asking them to lie down. Use your sleeping phrase, for example, "it's time to take your sleeping buddy and lie your head down on the pillow/mattress, close your eyes, it's time to sleep."
- You can occasionally pat, touch, sing, or hum for the first few nights to help your child fall asleep in their bed. Remember to try and reduce using this help so that it doesn't become their new sleep prop. Helping your child fall asleep is fine so you can offer comfort and guidance. But remember, this is just temporary help, as it is important that your child begins to fall asleep without needing extra help.
- If your child becomes upset, tell her that it's okay and you are here for her. You know it's tough right now, but they will soon know how to do this on their own. Give some guidance on what she can do. For example, laying her head down on the mattress and closing her eyes.
- If your child becomes very upset, you can pick her up to calm her after 30 minutes, but then she goes back to her bed again after a few minutes. *Take note! Do not do this if it makes your child more upset. This can lead to being overstimulated and then overtired. Don't hold your child too long so that they are becoming sleepy either.*
- Continue the above points until your child falls asleep.
- If you start seeing good improvements after three nights, you can move onto the next steps in Night 5 – 8.

⭐ **LEAVE & CHECK**
- Before you begin, choose a time that you'll start your checks. Choose between five to ten minutes.
- After a cuddle and your baby is beginning to get sleepy, but not too sleepy, put your baby into his crib.

- Say your sleeping phrase, tell your baby goodnight and that you'll see him in the morning.
- Leave the room. For the first few nights, stand outside of the door. Say your sleeping phrase from outside the door a few times if your child is upset. Let them know that you are still close by.
- Wait five to ten minutes before going back into the room to give them reassurance and comfort. Only use your voice and touch for comfort. After two minutes in the room, you'll say goodnight and then leave.
- You'll continue this until your child falls asleep.
- If your child becomes quiet, restart the time before going back in.

Crying

For any of these methods, if your child becomes upset, remember that this is a short-term tolerable stress and nothing that will harm him. Crying usually happens in a curve where it will become intense and hits a peak, but then reduces. If you don't see this, check in with yourself to see if you are interacting too much, as this will cause more frustration for your child. It's better to learn a new skill that takes a few days of hard work to set in a new life-long and healthier way of sleeping, rather than struggle for months on end with sleepless nights. The benefits of restful sleep will far outweigh the struggles of the first few nights.

Night waking

One piece of advice for night wakings is to have a plan on how you will respond. When we are woken in the middle of the night it's harder to stick to a plan. Therefore, write up a plan of action for night wakings, such as:

"When my child gets upset, I will ..."
- use the sleeping phrase for two minutes
- rub their back for two minutes
- pick up and hold my child for two minutes

"When my child wakes up at night, I will ..."
- wait for five minutes before going into her room
- listen to what my child's sounds are telling me
- use the plan of action for when my child gets upset

Your plan of action may look different but at least have a plan of how you will respond. Having a plan will help you stay on track!

Night waking guidance
- If it isn't an emergency, wait 10 minutes before you respond. This allows for time for your child to re-settle from a light stage of sleep and also learn that it's still night time.
- If you are not ready to begin with waiting 10 minutes, start with two minutes and increase the time each night by one minute.
- If you need to check in on your child, use the same strategy as bed-time. For example, if it's night 3, do the same method until your child falls asleep. Or for example, if it's night 8 on the fading method, you will sit in the chair by the door.
- If you have been feeding your child throughout the night, choose one to two times that you will feed her. You won't wait the 10 minutes before going in when you hear her wake. On the other wakings, use the same method you used at bedtime to help your child fall asleep.
- If you are feeding at night, be sure your child is actually hungry and not using this as help to go back to sleep.

Morning guidance
- Don't consider morning any time before your wake up time or at least not earlier than 6 am.
- Once it's time to get up, make a big deal about it being morning. Be sure to turn on lights or open the curtains to stimulate daytime in the body.
- Say good morning in a happy voice (even if you aren't feeling it!).
- Wait 10 minutes before feeding to delay the reason for waking. This also applies to cuddles in bed during the initial learning phase.

What you might see

As you are making new changes to your child's sleep, keep in mind that you might see some changes such as a little more crankiness, eating more or less, or sleepiness. I relate this to the same as when adults make big changes in their life. For example, think about when you started something new, like a new job. You were probably a bit stressed about the new adaptation and you didn't feel like yourself. You might have eaten more or less, been a little cranky due to the big change (or excited at first but then cranky after about a week or two), and sleepier. This type of change is not any different for your child! In fact, when your child starts daycare or preschool, you might notice them go through the same phases of change.

Is this the end of cuddles or co-sleeping?

This is a question I get asked often from parents wondering if they can ever co-sleep or cuddle with their baby in bed again. The answer is no, it's not the end! If you enjoy those things then just wait until your child is able to fall asleep more on their own before starting with morning cuddles or co-sleeping. This won't ruin anything if it's a night or morning here and there. If you do notice more night wakings, or early mornings, then start to reduce this again for a week to see if your child's sleep gets better again. If not, double check to see if you've started helping your child to fall asleep at night, added in a new prop, or if something big is changing for your child. This can include development leaps such as learning to crawl or walk, starting daycare or preschool, getting sick, or having an immunization.

Naptime – beginning on day 2

Daytime sleep is different from night time sleep, so keep in mind that naps (especially in cribs) might take more than two weeks to establish.

- After the nap routine (a shortened version of your bedtime routine. Example, snack, book, bed), put your child into the crib awake, again, without any sleep prop other than their sleeping buddy.
- Use the same strategies as the night before. For example, if you sat in the chair near the crib, that same process will be repeated.
- Try for 30 minutes. If your child hasn't slept, take a 10 minute break. You can leave the room with them and change their mindset. Look out the window or look at some pictures.
- After the break, go back to the room for a second try for 30 more minutes. You can have a quiet song while holding him, then put your child back in their bed.
- If your baby is under 12 months, you can use the stroller or a car ride for a nap instead.
- If your child won't sleep, skip that nap and try again at the next nap or bedtime. Have a quiet time together reading books if they seem overly sleepy. The next nap or bedtime can also be earlier by 20 to 30 minutes.

Short naps

If your child wakes up before an hour, go in quickly and try to coax them back to sleep with your sleeping phrase and gentle touch. If you've tried for 10 to 15 min to get them back to sleep with no success, then go ahead and get up. If this happens for the later nap time, then move bedtime 30 minutes earlier. The good news is that nap length improves with time! Most often naps will take longer than the nights to begin to fall into place. Stay consistent and keep trying!

If naps become difficult, it's okay to use a "free nap" time and go out with the stroller or a car ride for a nap. This is okay to do occasionally during this process because you also need to get through it! Try to keep this "free nap" only for every couple of days during the first two weeks. After your child begins to sleep better in her crib, then this can be used more often.

TIPS

I suggest that there be no toys in the crib, apart from your child's sleeping buddy. It is better to make the connection that the crib is for sleep and nothing else. An age appropriate pillow and blanket are okay.

Be as consistent as possible. This is crucial in helping your child sleep through the night and take naps on his own. It is a process that takes time, but it can also be a bit of a roller coaster ride for the first while. They may have a good night, then a not so good night, then a few good nights and so on. This is very normal and with time, it will become more and more consistent. Unless your child is sick, you should stick to your plan from now on.

If your child becomes sick during the plan, you would forgo the 10-minute wait period and respond when needed. Provide some comfort or a pain reliever, if needed, and then back into bed to drift off to sleep on their own again.

Night 5 through 8

You should start seeing ways that your child is able to fall asleep more on their own by night 5. What do you see them doing as they are falling asleep? Take a look at your sleep logs and see if you start to notice that your child might be able to fall asleep faster than the previous nights. Remember, small changes are signs that you are going in the right direction!

But wait!! You may also see some regression during these nights, but stick to your plan! It's common that your child may start to get used to the new changes but then test to see if this is really the way forward. Stay consistent and keep up the great work!

You may also start to have earlier wake ups and this is quite common and something that will disappear eventually. Your child is starting to sleep more at night and when he wakes up in the morning, he will feel rested and ready to go. Don't change anything and keep going. Early mornings may take a couple of weeks to disappear. To discourage early wakings, be sure to wait 10 minutes before feeding, playing, or anything that encourages getting up! See this as a good sign and that your child is sleeping more at night!

⭐ HOLD & HELP

- Not too many changes with this method during these nights. After a cuddle and your baby is beginning to get sleepy, put your baby in the crib, give him a little more time to settle on his own.
- You can help your baby to sleep with touch, gentle rocking while he lays there, singing, or using your sleeping phrase.
- If your baby becomes upset, wait one minute and then pick him up and help soothe for a couple of minutes before putting your baby back down.
- Repeat this process until your baby falls asleep.
- Start to notice if your baby can settle more on his own and doesn't need as much help to fall asleep.

⭐ FADING

- Move your chair further from your child's bed to about the middle of the room. You should start seeing her use some of her own ways to comfort herself for sleep. *If you have a small room and there isn't a "middle", be sure to move a bit further away and use less interaction with your child.*
- After the bedtime routine, put your child in her bed. Use less interaction on these nights but continue to use the sleeping phrase to help calm, if needed.
- If your child becomes very upset, occasionally go over and rub her back or help calm her in a way she prefers. Again, be aware if this causes her to become more upset. If so, do not use touch to help calm your child during this time.
- You will continue to sit in the room until your child falls asleep on her own.

⭐ LEAVE & CHECK

- Decide on the time that you will wait to go back in before you begin. It's best to extend the time from the previous nights.
- After a cuddle and your baby is beginning to get sleepy but not too sleepy, put your baby into his crib.
- Say your sleeping phrase, tell your baby goodnight and that you'll see them in the morning.
- Leave the room. Your child may not fuss as much and should be starting to fall asleep more on their own with fewer check-ins.
- Wait ten minutes before going back into the room to give him reassurance and comfort. After two minutes in the room, you'll say goodnight and then leave.

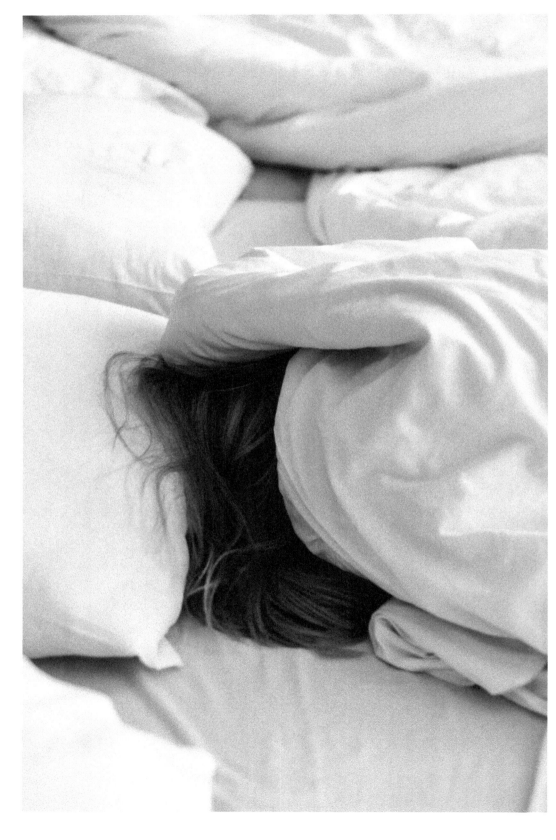

What about your sleep?

Alright, now that your child is starting to sleep better, let's talk about your sleep. It's just as important for you to get sleep too, so don't forget about yourself. It might be tempting to stay up late to finally have some time on your own, and do that sometimes, but the majority of the time it's wise to go to sleep at a reasonable time. Every sleep tip that I mention to use for your child will also work for you; have a bedtime routine, make sure your room is set up for sleep, and try to avoid using a screen before bedtime. Get a pair of blue light blocking glasses if you will be on a screen before bedtime. It won't fix your sleep completely, but it's better than nothing!

Remember, sleep is important for your mental and physical well-being! You'll be a better parent and partner for taking care of yourself.

Night 9 through 12

By this time you should be seeing some good progress! If you are not, double check that you have these factors checked off of the list:
- Awake window for your child's age (page 42)
- Bedroom environment (page 45)
- Your child's sleepy signs (page 41)
- Your child's ideal nap schedule for their age (page 117)
- Our day routines (page 53)
- Sign language that we'll use (page 100)
- Nap time routine (page 56)
- Bedtime routine (page 64)

Other factors that may play a role can include:
- Sleep regressions
- Developmental phases
- Immunizations
- Life changes – for example, starting daycare or preschool

Look over this list and see if you see anything that could cause some sleep disruptions. Give your child a few days and see if progress starts again.

This is also where temperament will play a big role! If you have a sensitive or spirited baby, you will need to keep having patience and stick with it or re-evaluate the method you are using.

If you are still struggling with going to sleep, make sure you aren't over stimulating your child. If they continue to get upset with your help, then it's not helping them. It would be better to do less in this situation.

If you are still struggling with night wakings, take a look at sleep props. Are you helping your child too much with falling asleep and he still needs your help at night?

⭐ HOLD & HELP

- By this time, you'll be helping your baby less. After a cuddle, put your baby into her crib, give her time to settle on her own.
- You can help your baby to sleep with touch, gentle rocking while she is laying down, singing or using your sleeping phrase. Start to reduce this help a little at a time. For example, if you were rocking or rubbing your baby's back, just keep your hand on them.
- If your baby becomes upset, pick them up and help soothe, but try to wait a little longer before picking them up.
- Repeat this process until your baby falls asleep.

⭐ FADING

- After you lay your child down, you'll sit by the door.
- Only use your sleeping phrases and gentle touch if needed.
- Your child will be developing his own strategies to fall asleep by this time. If not, double check the list at the top of this section.

⭐ LEAVE & CHECK

- After a cuddle, put your baby into their crib.
- Say your sleeping phrase, tell your baby goodnight and that you'll see her in the morning.
- Leave the room. Your child may not fuss as much and should be starting to fall asleep more on her own with fewer check-ins.
- Wait 10 to 15 minutes before going back into the room to give her reassurance and comfort. After a two minutes in the room, you'll say goodnight and then leave.

- By this time you'll probably start to hear the difference between a help cry, an annoyed cry, and a stubborn cry. If not, try to listen to the difference between the cries and take notes as to what works with each cry.

Night 13 and 14

You're doing amazing! You should be starting to see some changes by now. Be sure to look at your sleep logs and compare Night 1 to tonight!

⭐ HOLD & HELP
- You'll continue as the last couple of nights. After a cuddle, put your baby into his crib and give him time to settle on his own.
- You can help your baby to sleep with touch, gentle rocking while they are laying down, singing or using your sleeping phrase. Start to reduce this help a little at a time. For example, keeping your hand on him, then start removing your hand more and more when he is calm.
- If your baby becomes upset, pick him up and help soothe, but try to wait a little longer before picking him up again.
- Repeat this process until your baby falls asleep. You'll continue this process until your baby starts falling asleep on his own after laying them down.

⭐ FADING
- After you lay your child down, say good night, help calm for a minute or two, if needed, then leave the room.
- You'll stay just outside of the door to help calm with your sleeping phrase, if needed.
- Try to listen to their sounds. Do they become quiet? Good!
- If your baby cries longer than 10 minutes, you can go back into the room for two minutes, say your sleeping phrase, use some touch if that helps calm them, and then leave again. Repeat every 10 minutes if necessary.

If you child is having a hard time falling asleep by night 12 through 14, double check the checklist on page 187. Some temperaments will take longer to adjust or if your baby is in a sleep regression or developmental leap.

⭐ **LEAVE & CHECK**
- After a cuddle, put your baby into her crib.
- Say your sleeping phrase, tell your baby goodnight and that you'll see her in the morning.
- Leave the room. Your child may not fuss as much and should be starting to fall asleep more on their own with fewer check-ins.
- Wait 10 to 15 minutes before going back into the room to give them reassurance and comfort. After a two minutes in the room, you'll say goodnight and then leave again.
- You'll continue this until your child can fall asleep more and more on their own without check-ins.

Happy sleep and beyond!

⭐ **HOLD & HELP**
- You'll continue as the last couple of nights but it's important to keep reducing the time you help your baby fall asleep.
- After a cuddle, put your baby into his crib and give him time to settle on his own.
- You can help your baby to sleep with touch, gentle rocking while they are laying down, singing or using your sleeping phrase.
- If your baby becomes upset, pick him up and help soothe, but try to wait a little longer before picking him up each time.
- Repeat this process until your baby falls asleep. You'll continue this process until your baby starts falling asleep on his own after laying them down.

- The most important thing to remember with this method is that you need to reduce the amount of help you provide while your child is falling asleep.

⭐ FADING
- After night 14, you lay your child down, say good night (help calm for a minute or two, if needed), then leave the room.
- If your baby cries longer than 10 minutes, you can go back into the room for two minutes, say your sleeping phrase, use some touch if that helps calm them, and then leave again. Repeat every 10 minutes if necessary.
- You will understand your child's sounds and movements now and know when and how they fall asleep.

⭐ LEAVE & CHECK
- After a cuddle, put your baby into her crib.
- Say your sleeping phrase, tell your baby goodnight and that you'll see her in the morning.
- Leave the room. Your child may not fuss as much and should be starting to fall asleep more on their own with fewer check-ins.
- Wait 10 to 15 minutes before going back into the room to give reassurance and comfort. After a two minutes in the room, you'll say goodnight and then leave again.
- You'll continue this until your child can fall asleep more and more on their own without check-ins.

Congratulations on completing your sleep method and giving your child the gift of healthy sleep habits for life! While you might not be fully finished with making changes, think back to just two weeks ago and how your child was (not) sleeping. Be sure to celebrate the success!

Sleep trouble checklist

– a longer version if you are having trouble

If you are having trouble through the plan then take a look at this list to see if you have areas to change or work on.

Awake windows
Is your child having to push past their awake window? This could be causing overtiredness.

Naps
Is your child having too many or too long of naps and isn't tired at bedtime?

Day time routines
Do you have consistent routines in place for your child?

Bedtime routine
Getting sleepy during any of the routines? Work on keeping your child awake during the feeding or routine. Try moving the routine a little earlier or feeding where your child stays awake, on the couch with lights on, for example.

Room environment
Is it dark, cool, and quiet?

Consistency
Are you responding to your child in a consistent way?

Sleep props
Is your child still needing a prop to help fall asleep?

Teething
Generally teething pain might last a day or two. Is there a leap or something else your child is going through?

Milestones or regressions
Is your child in a leap or regression stage?

Other possible factors:
- Immunizations
- Tags in clothing
- Itchy skin
- Injuries that make it hard to sleep

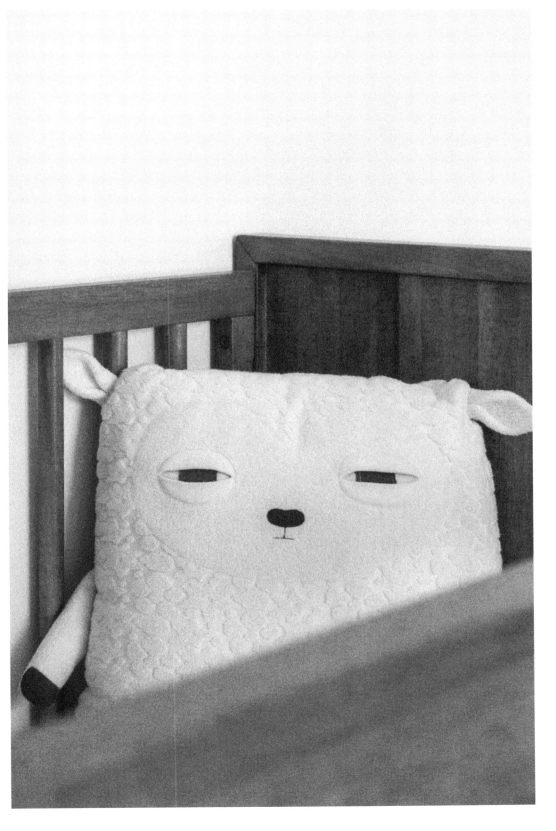

Appendix

Within this section you can download the sleep logs and bedtime routine chart at HappySleepingBaby.com/extras

Setting up for sleep checklist

Here's a checklist to help you put together a plan for your family.
- Bedroom environment (page 42)
- Awake window for your child's age (page 45)
- Your child's sleepy signs (page 41)
- Your child's ideal nap schedule for their age (page 117)
- Our day routines (page 53)
- Sign language that we'll use (page 100)
- Nap time routine (page 56)
- Bedtime routine (page 64)

Sleep and nap chart

Age (months)	General awake window between naps	Daily sleep requirements	Number of naps	Wake if nap is longer than
Newborn	45 min – 1 hour	14 – 19 hours	3 – 5	3 hours
3 – 6	1.5 – 2 hours	13 – 16 hours	3 – 4	2 – 3 hours
6 – 13	2.5 – 3.5 hours	12 – 16 hours	2 – 3	2 – 2.5 hours
12 – 3 yrs	4 – 6 hours	11 – 14 hours	1	2 hours

Sleep logs

Use the sleep logs to keep track of how sleep changes are going for your family. You can see patterns for sleep or habits for your child using the sleep logs. You should start seeing changes to sleep within a few days, and remember that small changes are changes in the right direction!

You can also download sleep log templates at HappySleepingBaby.com/extras

Happy Sleep Log

Week	Monday	Tuesday	Wednesday	Thursday	Friday	Saturday	Sunday
Wake up time							
Activity							
1st nap time							
Result and time it took to sleep							
Nap length							
2nd nap time							
Result and time it took to sleep							
Nap length							
3rd nap time							
Result and time it took to sleep							
Nap length							
4th nap time							
Result and time it took to sleep							
Nap length							
Bedtime routine							
In bed time							
Result and time it took to sleep							
Night wakings?							
Time/duration							
Time/duration							
Time/duration							
Notes:							

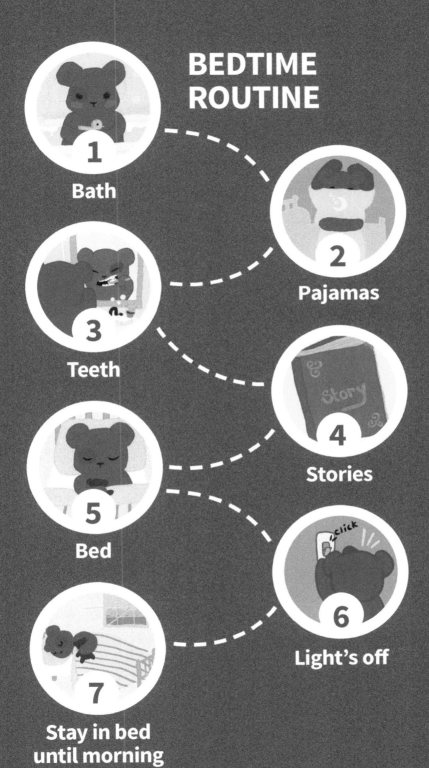

BEDTIME ROUTINE

1 Bath

2 Pajamas

3 Teeth

4 Stories

5 Bed

6 Light's off

7 Stay in bed until morning

Hold & help sleep plan cheat sheet

Use sleep logs to track progress

Our sleep goals:

Our sleeping phrase:

Our night waking plan:

Nights 1 through 4 – holding baby

- After a cuddle and your baby is beginning to get sleepy, put your baby into his crib, give him some time to settle on his own.
- You can help your baby to sleep with touch, gentle rocking while they are laying down, singing or using your sleeping phrase.
- If your baby becomes upset, pick him up and help soothe.
- Repeat this process until your baby falls asleep.

Nights 5 through 8 – holding baby, putting down more

- Use the same process as nights 1 w– 4 but work on putting your baby down more often and trying to soothe in his crib.
- You can help your baby to sleep with touch, gentle rocking while he lays there, singing, or using your sleeping phrase.
- Start to notice if your baby can settle more on his own and doesn't need as much help to fall asleep.

Around nights 4 through 6

Sometimes a child will start adapting to the changes and then around night 4, 5, or 6 they will test the boundaries with you. Don't change anything and continue on being consistent with your changes.

Nights 9 through 12 – holding baby, putting down more

- You'll be helping your baby less to fall asleep.
- After a cuddle, put your baby into his crib, give him time to settle on his own.
- You can help your baby to sleep with touch, gentle rocking while he is laying down, singing or using your sleeping phrase. Start to reduce this help a little at a time.
- If your baby becomes upset, pick him up and help soothe, but try to wait a little longer before picking him up.
- Repeat this process until your baby falls asleep.

Nights 13 & 14 – holding baby, putting down more

- After a cuddle, put your baby into his crib and give him time to settle on his own.
- Work on reducing how much you help your baby to sleep with touch, gentle rocking while they are laying down, singing or using your sleeping phrase.
- If your baby becomes upset, pick him up and help soothe, but try to wait a little longer before picking him up again.
- Repeat this process until your baby falls asleep.
- You'll continue this process until your baby starts falling asleep on his own after laying him down.

Night 14 and beyond!

You'll continue as the last couple of nights but it's important to keep reducing the time you help your baby fall asleep.

Fading sleep plan cheat sheet

Use sleep logs to track progress

Our sleep goals:

Our sleeping phrase:

Our night waking plan:

Nights 1 through 4 – sitting beside the crib
- Sit beside the crib but not facing your child.
- Say your key phrase – every 2 – 3 minutes maximum, only if needed.
- Use gentle touch – 30 seconds to one minute maximum.
- Do all this until your child falls asleep. No time limit.
- Use the phrase or use touch occasionally to help calm down. But we do not want this to become a new prop.
- Help lay down five times, after five times, give reminders to lay down.

Nights 5 through 8 – sitting in the middle of the room
- Use less interaction on these nights but continue to use your sleeping phrase.
- Stay in your chair as much as possible!
- If your child is very upset, occasionally use gentle touch.
- Continue to sit in the room until your child falls asleep on their own.

Around nights 4 through 6
Sometimes a child will start adapting well to the changes and then around night 4, 5, or 6 they will test the boundaries with you. Don't change anything and continue on being consistent with your changes.

Nights 9 through 12 – sitting by the door
- Only use the sleeping phrase and gentle touch, if needed.
- Your child will be developing his own strategies to fall asleep by this time.

Nights 13 & 14 – outside the door
- No longer in the room but outside the door using your sleeping phrase, if needed.
- If your child cries longer than 10 minutes, go in, use a sleeping phrase, gentle touch, and leave the room.
- Repeat every 10 minutes, if needed.

Night 14 and beyond!
- No longer in the room.
- If your baby cries longer than 10 minutes, go in, use a sleeping phrase, gentle touch, and leave the room.
- Repeat every 10 minutes, if needed, but you should understand and know your child's sounds and how they go to sleep now!

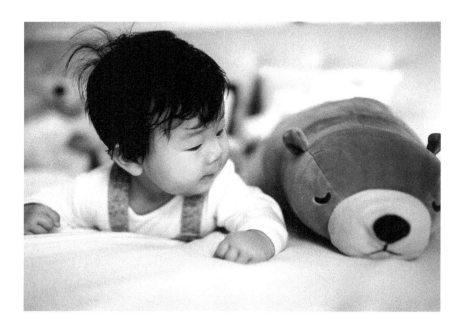

Leave & check sleep plan cheat sheet

Use sleep logs to track progress

Our sleep goals:

Our sleeping phrase:

Our night waking plan:

Nights 1 through 4 – outside the door
- After a cuddle, put your baby into her crib.
- Say your sleeping phrase, tell your baby goodnight and that you'll see her in the morning.
- Leave the room but stand next to the door. Say your sleeping phrase to help calm and assure your child.
- Wait five to ten minutes before going back into the room to give them reassurance and comfort.
- After a two minutes in the room, you'll say goodnight and then leave.
- You'll continue this until your child falls asleep.

Nights 5 through 8 – outside the door
- Repeat the same process as nights 1 – 4.
- Reduce the number of times you use your sleeping phrase.
- Wait a little longer before going into the room to help comfort.

Around Nights 4 through 6
Sometimes a child will start adapting well to the changes and then around night 4, 5, or 6 they will test the boundaries with you. Don't change anything and continue on being consistent with your changes.

Nights 9 through 12 – outside the door, if needed
- Only use the sleeping phrase and go into the room if needed.
- Your child will be developing her own strategies to fall asleep by this time

Nights 13 & 14 – outside the door, if needed
- Only go into the room if your child cries longer than 10 to 15 minutes.
- If your child starts to become quiet, let her be for a little bit and see if she can calm herself.

Night 14 and beyond!
- If your baby cries longer than 10 to 15 minutes, go in, use a sleeping phrase, gentle touch, and leave the room.
- Repeat, if needed, but you should understand and know your child's sounds and how they go to sleep now!

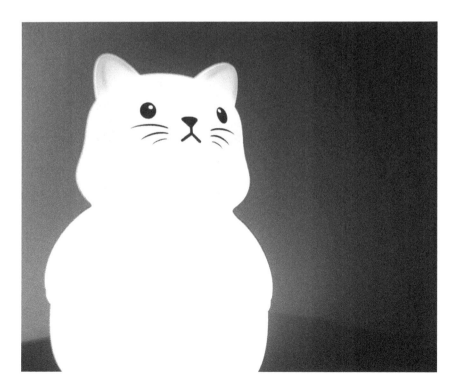

Notes

Notes

Notes

References

American Academy of Pediatrics. (2020). *Healthy Sleep Habits: How Many Hours Does Your Child Need?* Retrieved from: https://www.healthychildren.org/English/healthy-living/sleep/Pages/healthy-sleep-habits-how-many-hours-does-your-child-need.aspx

American Academy of Pediatrics. (2020). *Safe Sleep.* Retrieved from: https://www.aap.org/en-us/about-the-aap/aap-press-room/campaigns/Safe-Sleep/Pages/default.aspx

American Academy of Pediatrics. (2020). *Sleep.* Retrieved from: https://www.healthychildren.org/English/healthy-living/sleep/Pages/default.aspx

Aron, E.N. PhD. (2002). *The Highly Sensitive Child: Helping our children thrive when the world overwhelms them.* Harmony Books. New York.

Babysleepscience.com (2020). *Baby Sleep Science Mini Blog: Teething.* Retrieved from: https://www.babysleepscience.com/single-post/2014/06/12/*baby-sleep-science-mini-blog-teething*

Babysleepscience.com (2020). Naps 101 (Part 4): *When and How Will My Baby Drop Naps?* Retrieved from: https://www.babysleepscience.com/single-post/2014/03/25/nap-101-part-4-when-and-how-will-my-baby-drop-naps

Babysleepsite.com. (2020). *Sample Baby Sleep & Feeding Schedules.* Retrieved from: https://www.babysleepsite.com/baby-sleep-feeding-schedules/

Barr, M. (2020). *What is the Period of PURPLE Crying?* Retrieved from: http://purplecrying.info/what-is-the-period-of-purple-crying.php#

Briant, M.Z. (2011). *Baby Sign Language Basics*. Hayu House, Inc.

Bryson, T.P. PhD. (2020). *The Bottom Line for Baby*. Ballantine Books. New Tork.

Boyce, W.T. MD. (2019). *The Orchid and The Dandelion*. Alfred A. Knopf. New York.

Center on the Developing Child at Harvard University (2020). *Building the Brain's "Air Traffic Control" System: How Early Experiences Shape the Development of Executive Function: Working Paper No. 11*. Retrieved from: www.developingchild.harvard.edu.

Center on the Developing Child, Harvard University. (2020). *Early Childhood Mental Health*. Retrieved from: http://developingchild.harvard. edu/science/deep-dives/mental-health

Center on the Developing Child at Harvard University (2020). *Enhancing and Practicing Executive Function Skills with Children from Infancy to Adolescence*. Retrieved from: www.developingchild.harvard.edu.

Center on the Developing Child at Harvard University. (2020). *Executive function and self-regulation*. Retrieved from: https://developingchild. harvard.edu/science/key-concepts/executive-function/

Center on the Developing Child at Harvard University. (2020). *Toxic Stress*. Retrieved from: https://developingchild.harvard.edu/science/ key-concepts/toxic-stress/

Clear, J. (2020). *40 Years of Stanford Research Found That People With This One Quality Are More Likely to Succeed*. Retrieved from: https://jamesclear.com/delayed-gratification

Cleveland Clinic. (2020). *Sleep Basics*. Retrieved from: https://my.clevelandclinic.org/health/articles/12148-sleep-basics

Conti, R. (2019). *Delay of gratification*. Retrieved from: https://www.britannica.com/science/delay-of-gratification#ref1206154

Dement, W.C. (1999) *The Promise of Sleep*. New York, New York. Dell Publishing.

Dewar, G. Ph.D. (2018). *What's normal? An evidence-based baby sleep chart*. Retrieved from: https://www.parentingscience.com/baby-sleep-chart.html

Duhigg, C. (NA). *The Power of Habit: Why We Do What We Do, and How to Change*. Kindle Edition.

Dunstan Baby. (2020). *Inside the Seminar: Priscilla Teaches New Mothers the Dunstan Baby Language*. Retrieved from: https://www.youtube.com/watch?v=9zSajTrCnKs

Feber, R. M.D. (2006). *Solve your Child's Sleep Problems: Revised Edition*. Fireside. New York, New York.

Firstfiveyears.org. (2019). *Why spend one-on-one time with your child*. Retrieved from: https://www.firstfiveyears.org.au/child-development/why-spend-oneonone-time-with-your-child

Flynn-Evans, E. PhD. MPH., and Casano, M. BSN. MA. (2016). *Baby Sleep Science Guide*.

Galland, B.C., Taylor, B.J., Elder, D.E., Herbison, P. (2011) *Normal sleep patterns in infants and children: a systematic review of observational studies*. PMID: 21784676, DOI: 10.1016/j.smrv.2011.06.001

Harvard Health. (2020). *The fourth trimester: What you should know*. Retrieved from: https://www.health.harvard.edu/blog/the-fourth-trimester-what-you-should-know-2019071617314

Hogg, T & Blau, M. (2001). *Secrets of the Baby Whisperer.* New York. Ballantine Publishing Group.

Hogg, T & Blau, M. (2002). *Secrets of the Baby Whisperer for Toddlers.* NewYork. Ballantine Publishing Group.

Hogg, T & Blau, M. (2005). *The Baby Whisperer Solves all your Problems.* NewYork, New York. Atria Books.

Infant Mental Health Community Training Institute. (2016). Online web courses from Infant Mental Health Promotion. Toronto, Canada.

Iwata, S. et al. (2017). *Dependence of nighttime sleep duration in one-month-old infants on alterations in natural and artificial photoperiod.* PMCID: PMC5355994. DOI: 10.1038/srep44749

Karp, H. M.D. (2003). *The Happiest Baby on the Block.* New York, New York. Bantam Bell.

Karp, H. M.D. (2016). *Happiest Baby Q&A: How much jiggly motion is safe with my baby?* Retrieved from: https://www.youtube.com/watch?v=sB-2Fw3MFlhk

KidsHealth.org. Reviewed by Ben-joseph, E.P. M.D. (2017). *Night Terrors.* Retrieved from: https://kidshealth.org/en/parents/terrors.html

Kohn, A. (2005). *Unconditional Parenting.* NewYork, New York. Atria Books.

Kurcinka, M.S. (NA). *Kids, Parents, and Power Struggles.* HarperCollins e-books.

Kurcinka, M.S. (2006). *Raising Your Spirited Child, Rev. ed.* New York: Harper.

Kurcinka, M.S. (NA). *Sleepless in America – Is your child misbehaving or missing sleep?* HarperCollins e-books.

Kutner, L. (Ph.D). (2016). *What's Your Baby's Temperament?* Retrieved from http://psychcentral.com/lib/whats-your-babys-temperament/

Lewis, M.D. PhD. and Granic, I. PhD. (NA). *Bed Timing - The "when-to" guide to helping your child sleep.* HarperCollins e-books.

Medina, J. (2014) *Brain Rules for Baby: How to Raise a Smart and Happy Child from Zero to Five.* Seattle, Washington. Pear Press.

Meltzer, L.J. and McLaughlin Crabtree, V. (2015). *Pediatric Sleep Problems – A Clinician's Guide to Behavioral Interventions.* Washington, D.C. American Psychological Association.

Mindell, J.A. PhD. (NA). *Sleeping Through the Night* (Revised Edition). HarperCollins eBooks.

Mindell, J.A. PhD., & Owens, J.A. (2015). *A Clinical Guide to Pediatric Sleep: diagnosis and management of sleep problems.* Philadelphia, PA. Wolters Kluwer.

Moody, E. D.D.S. (2020). *Teething 101: Tips from a Dentist and Dad.* Retrieved from: https://mouthmonsters.mychildrensteeth.org/teething-101-tips-from-a-dentist-and-dad/

National Center for Biotechnology Information. (1996). *Physiology of growth hormone secretion during sleep.* Retrieved from: https://www.ncbi.nlm.nih.gov/pubmed/8627466

National Sleep Foundation (2015). *National Sleep Foundation Recommends New Sleep Times.* Retrieved from: https://www.sleepfoundation.org/press-release/national-sleep-foundation-recommends-new-sleep-times

National Sleep Foundation (2019). *Sleep drive and your body clock.* Retrieved online from: https://www.sleepfoundation.org/sleep-topics/sleep-drive-and-your-body-clock

National Institutes of Health. (2018). *Sleep deprivation increases Alzheimer's protein.* Retrieved from: https://www.nih.gov/news-events/nih-research-matters/sleep-deprivation-increases- alzheimers-protein

National Institutes of Health. (2018). *How Sleep Clears the Brain.* Retrieved online from: https://www.nih.gov/news-events/nih-research-matters/how-sleep-clears-brain

Plas, X. & Plooij, F. (2017) *The Wonder Weeks Milestone Guide.* The Netherlands, Kiddy Publishing.

Pregnancy, Birth, and Baby. (2020). *What is the fourth trimester?* Retrieved from: https://www.pregnancybirthbaby.org.au/blog/what-is-the-fourth-trimester

Price, A.M.H., Wake, M., Ukoumunne, O. & Hiscock, H. (2012). *Five-Year Follow-up of Harms and Benefits of Behavioral Infant Sleep Intervention: Randomized Trial.* Pediatrics October 2012, 130 (4) 643-651; DOI: https://doi.org/10.1542/peds.2011-3467

Raising Children. (2020). *2–3 Years: Toddler Development.* Retrieved from: https://raisingchildren.net.au/toddlers/development/development-tracker-1-3-years/2-3-years

ScienceDirect.com. (2018) *Beta-Amyloid.* Retrieved online from: https://www.sciencedirect.com/topics/neuroscience/beta-amyloid

Siegel, D.J. M.D., & Bryson, T.P. PhD. (2011). The Whole Brain Child. Delacorte Press. New York.

Shoda, Y., Mischel, W., & Peake, P.K. (1990). *"Predicting Adolescent Cognitive and Self-Regulatory Competencies from Preschool Delay of Gratification: Identifying Diagnostic Conditions"* (PDF). Developmental Psychology. 26 (6): 978–986. doi:10.1037/0012-1649.26.6.978. Archived from the original (PDF) on October 4, 2011.

Sleepfoundation.org. (2020). *Night Terrors.* Retrieved online from: https://www.sleepfoundation.org/articles/3-ways-tell-nightmare-night-terror

Sleepfoundation.org. (2020). *What is White Noise?* Retrieved from: https://www.sleepfoundation.org/bedroom-environment/white-noise

Sleep Sense. (2014). *Baby Sleep Training Certification.* In-person training.

Spencer Institute. (2017). *Sleep Science Coach Certification.* Online course material.

Stanford Children's Health. (2017). *Newborn Sleep Patterns.* Retrieved online from: https://www.stanfordchildrens.org/en/topic/default?id=newborn-sleep-patterns

The Child Sleep Institute. (2019). *Sleeposium 2019.* Online summit.

The Child Sleep Institute. (2020). *Sleeposium 2020.* Online summit.

The Health Sciences Academy. (2020). Advanced Child and Brain Development Nutritional Advisor Certification.

Tough, P. (2012). *How Children Succeed: Grit, Curiosity, and the Hidden Power of Character.* Houghton Mifflin Harcourt Publishing Company. New York, New York.

Tuck.com. (2019). *Stages of sleep and sleep cycles*. Retrieved from: https://www.tuck.com/stages/

Walker, M. (2018) *Why We Sleep – The New Science of Sleep and Dreams*. Penguin Random House UK.

WebMD.com (2020). *How to Talk to Your Baby*. Retrieved from: https://www.webmd.com/parenting/baby/baby-talk-language#1

Weissbluth, M. M.D. (2015). *Healthy Sleep Habits, Happy Child. Fourth Edition*. Ballantine Books. New York.

Wikipedia.org (2020). *Stanford Marshmallow Experiment*. Retrieved from: https://en.wikipedia.org/wiki/Stanford_marshmallow_experiment

Yogman, M., et al. (2018). *The Power of Play: A Pediatric Role in Enhancing Development in Young Children*. Pediatrics. 142 (3) e20182058; DOI: 10.1542/peds.2018-2058. Retrieved from: https://pediatrics.aappublications.org/content/142/3/e20182058

Zhoua, J., et al. (2012). *Pink noise: Effect on complexity synchronization of brain activity and sleep consolidation*. Journal of Theoretical Biology, Volume 306, 7 August 2012, Pages 68-72. Retrieved from: https://www.sciencedirect.com/science/article/abs/pii/S0022519312001798

Thank you...

To my husband for believing in me and sticking with me when nights and days were long, both with our daughter and through the process of writing this book!

To my little sweet pea who went through this time with me and turned life into a wonderful journey!

To Katti for her wonderful design, to Andrea for helping to organize my material, to Judi for editing, and to Polya for her relationship advice.

To each family who has put trust in me and taught me so much with each experience with their family!